Self♥Love
Potions

Self♥Love Potions

An Herbalist's Perspective on Love and Self Healing

Cynthia Hartson

Writers Advantage
New York   Lincoln   Shanghai

Self♥Love Potions
An Herbalist's Perspective on Love and Self Healing

Writers Advantage
an imprint of iUniverse, Inc.

For information address:
iUniverse
2021 Pine Lake Road, Suite 100
Lincoln, NE 68512
www.iuniverse.com

ISBN: 0-595-23935-8

Printed in the United States of America

I dedicate this book to my daughter
❤ *Amber Mae.*
Know you are loved, unconditionally, for all eternity.
*Thank you for all you are and for all the little things you do that are just
between you and God. I can't wait to spend an eternity with you in
heaven, but while you are here,
may this book encourage you.*

∼

*I also dedicate this book
to the next generation of healers,
my students and the people that loved me
before I could love myself*❤

~ A Glimpse ~

♥Last night, something in the air caught my attention. I can't say for sure, but it was as if I could feel God's reassuring breath upon my neck as I typed pages into my book. I sat quiet for a moment, my balcony doors open to the sound of the ocean's evening routine.

The curtains danced to the flicker a of dozen peppermint candles, which lined my open window's sill. I caught a glimpse of the sun's trailing children, chasing her over the horizon, as she called out her amber-colored curfew. I drew in a deep breath and smiled to myself.

Take a moment, my heart spoke to me.

I followed these words out onto the balcony, where I was greeted by the demanding droop of abundance from an unattended herb basket. I obliged with necessary pruning, while enjoying the playful sprinkling from my Guardian Angel fountain, her constant flow of water soothing my evening dreams. As the aroma of cut herbs filled the air, once again I felt it:

Take a moment.

There was a warm kiss of ocean in the air. As if drawn by a familiar potion, my head was guided toward the starlit sky. I gave my trusting body to the down pillows that lined the lounge chair, falling safely and contentedly into that moment. I blew the hair from my eyes, with hopes that the picture my heart was pounding into the night would reveal itself more clearly. With each breath I was filled; in each blink I became more aware; each pulse pushed the feeling closer to the surface of my tingling skin; and, suddenly, I understood the message the night air was pouring over me. I took a "moment" and this was revealed:

> *It is the honest interest in life's 'moments' that keep the Spirit and mind in harmony. It is within these moments that we understand the emotionally healing nature of faith, the physically destructive nature of fear, and the curative value of family and friendship. Powerful ingredients necessary to create a Self♥Loving Potion are found within these faith-filled moments. Take this moment in time to discover them!*

Giggling, I pulled my knees, along with a pillow, closer in to my chest. I felt full of life, full in the moment, full with inspiration.

I have a need to share my perspective of life's "moments," to the best of my ability to do so, with all who will listen.

So my friends, in my honest attempt to share a few of my moments with you, may I ask that you *take a moment,* too. A moment for your God, for your family, for your friends, and for yourself. I pray that, in these moments, your own unique Self♥Love Potion will be revealed to you. ♥

~ Warmly,
Cynthia♥Hartson~
Laguna Niguel, California.

♥ Acknowledgments

♥ My beloved Grandma Dracoules, who was always satisfied with me, no matter what I had done. Her steadfast unconditional love gave me extraordinary courage to live out loud. Thank you Grammy, for your many gifts of healing and for giving me my faith.

♥ My mother, Beverly, and stepfather, Ray—what an awesome task being a parent is. Thank you for taking the adventure, together.

♥ My little brother, Bryan, his wife Patricia, and my two beautiful nieces, thank you for sharing your light and life with me, and for giving me opportunity to share mine with you. I love you.

♥ My big brother, Jerry, wife Sandy, and nephew, JJ, thank you for holding my world together at a time when I could not even figure out how to breathe. You are such an important part of my living.

♥ Amber's godfather, Jim. You are a stalwart example of a Christian man dedicated to his family. For this, through the eyes of my daughter, I am forever grateful.

♥ Rene, you've been the light in the darkness of many gloomy nights. Thank you for your true and rich friendship, hours of Spiritual counseling, and the timely gift of Heather.

♥ Steve, thank you for breaking my heart wide open, which allowed me to dance to the beautiful music hidden inside.

♥ Tina, may the laughter never end. You are a cherished sister in Christ and the spirit of this life! Mwahhhhh! I love you darlin'! See yer l'il face in forever!

♥ Channel, Tony, Dillon, Devin, and Dominick, thank you for the moments, which are too many to count. You give me hope.

♥ Melissa, thank you for going the distance with me. You're a rare and cherished friend!

♥ Miss Judy Rose, I could not have done what I did, if you didn't do what you do. Thank you for your courage, from the bottom of my heart.

♥ Dr. Jensen and Marie, thank you for your encouragement, honesty, and guidance over the years. The twinkle in your eye was all that ever mattered, and working alongside of you was the greatest experience of my life. See you when I get there.

♥ My Canadian Gal Pal, Annette, I am forever grateful for your friendship and hospitality. Thank you for tending my broken wings and insisting I fly with the eagles. Look, I'm flying!

♥ Rosemarie, my faithful guardian angel. Eternal thanks for remembering the little things, and promises kept between cherubs.

♥ Dr. Dave and Helen, your faith in God is awe-inspiring. Thank you for the prayers at a time when nothing else mattered.

♥ Kevin, you are my living proof that God's power is made great in our weaknesses. Thank you for being an extension of God's love in my life. I love your integrity!

♥ Mara, thank you for your many gifts of love and time. You are precious!

♥ Wordman, as a writer's inspiration, you will remain "always" in my prayers.

♥ Dan, thank you for sharing so much of yourself and so many beautiful moments with me. I pray God will always lead you by the path which He knows is best for your life. He knows better than we do. Be faithful to Him.

♥ My friends, Alex, Amanda, Barbara, Beverly, Darryl, Don, Dusty, Ed, Jeannette, Karen, Katie, Mark, Mary-Jane, Mike, Rocio, Tara, and Michelle. Some moments larger and longer than others, yet, with each and every one of them come the inspiration and the words. Thank you.

♥

And finally,

♥ To an inspiring business partner and a dear, respected, cherished friend, ♥ Michael. You are a wonderfully loving man of God. As I've observed your healing touch change the lives of so many people, I have become conscious that your sincere devotion to that which is good and right has also changed mine. Thank you for demanding that I do my very best and for persistently striving to create a positive environment in which I can enthusiastically serve God and my life's purpose. How can, "Thank you," be adequate to express my gratitude for the countless hours you have spent painstakingly editing my misspelled words? Your reliability is a gift I shall ever cherish. My life has been blessed by the knowing of you, and I am honored to call you my friend! You have helped me to find my own Kenya, and I thank you for allowing me to participate in the realization of yours. Sometimes, there just aren't enough words, or adequate ones, to express what the heart already knows, come what may.

Any work is a cooperative effort and there are many more to thank. If I have not done so with words, I have in my prayers, and I thank God every day for your blessings in my life. ♥

Note:
Self♥Love Potions is not intended as medical advice. It is meant to enlighten the reader, inspire, and offer interpretations derived from an already existing body of sacred wisdom. ♥

Please consult a health professional to assist you with the healing you require.

I hope this book will light the way.

♥ Contents ♥

PART One

Chapter One

Chapter One

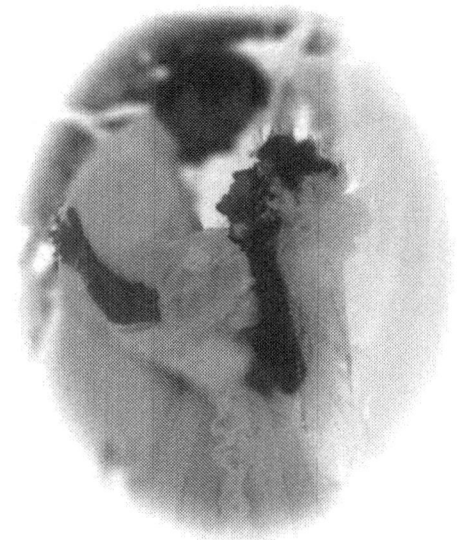

♥ A Loving Voice

Those Days may be over…but more importantly, you are free to be loved. Before you depart this world, you will know that you were absolutely and utterly loved…as God had always intended.

~ Enchanted

Enchanted by forever-after, she had been in love with love from the very beginning. Her cup of life was full in anticipation of a devoted man. She danced and delighted to the tune of love's promise— its purity and sweet nature.

The thirsting in man's hardened heart eagerly consumed her charm, and, as her promise was shattered, what was once a carefree Spirit became a timid believer. Yet, she persisted in the dance, a self-made muse.

With little to offer from an empty cup, she realized she could no longer serve the thirsting in man's heart. All she had left was her faith.

It was then, at that moment, that she released her empty cup back to the heavens. High above her head the cup sailed, soaring toward its lender.

Instead of the Spirit refilling the cup with enchantment, the Spirit filled the woman with grace.

The young girl, who in the beginning had been in love with love, began dancing and delighting once again to the promise and sweetness of nature. Only this time, she was dancing to the tune of faith, eternally full from within.

~C

The Fundamental Ingredient
Spirituality

♥ Yes, I realize that asking you to investigate or create a "Spirituality" recipe may freak some of you out straight away. You may even consider putting this book down altogether, right now, because of some preconceived idea of what you think I mean by that word. However, I encourage you to hang in there for these first few pages. You will get a better picture of what I am suggesting if you give me a few chapters to plant the words it into simple stories for you.

See, I believe with all my heart, that Spirituality is the single most important ingredient when it comes to developing an intimately healing Self♥Loving recipe. It's a bold statement, I know, and, conventionally speaking, you might require that I have a more liturgical credential than I possess before you take that statement to heart. But the truth is the truth—no matter how you slice it up or who serves it to you—and I believe that statement to be true, with every fiber of my being.

I'm not necessarily talking about acts of religion (although I am proud of being a Christian, which allows me to draw upon those acts for my own potions), but what I am speaking of here is: your belief system, your self-worth, hope, and trust.

> ♥ The connection between heaven and earth, and your footing within that space. ♥

My wish is that you will appreciate the importance of Spiritual healing and Spiritual Se_f♥Love on a very personal level by the time you finish reading this book. Even if the word "Spirituality" scares you to pieces right now, please keep reading, anyway. You just may find you'll want to add this very important ingredient to your future Self♥Love recipe, in massive doses. Know this: it will always be your choice!

♥ As a naturopath and herbalist, I see many physical health issues arise out of life's daily emotional stresses. A lack of faith can trickle into many areas of our lives, including:

   ♥ money issues,
   ♥ jobs,
   ♥ family,
   ♥ relationships,
   ♥ and certainly, Self♥Love.

This, in turn, can create feelings of loss, frustration, misfortune, and what I like to refer to as the "Why Me?" syndrome. I know because I've been there.

Today, I am frequently asked where I've acquired the positive attitude (faith) that tomorrow can always be better than today. You know what I believe? I believe that today will always "lead" to a better tomorrow (regardless of how I might feel in the moment), because I have this sense that I am, today, exactly where I am supposed to be, first by my choices, then by a bigger, perfect plan. See, when I lean on my faith, I am trusting that the choices I've made in my life will be used for a larger, perfect plan by a greater consciousness than my own, no matter how poor my past choices may have been.

> ♥ From my choices to a bigger, perfect plan. ♥

It comes from that sense of connection between heaven and earth that I was talking about. It's not always easy for me to keep my chin up and have faith in the tough times, though. Trust me, there were times when I would cry out, even in my sleep! Even today, although it appears most of my heartbreaks have diminished, and it feels as if I am moving in a direction of peace and abundance in the areas in which I was once struggling, there are still times when someone I love, or a family member of someone I love, will say or do something so mean, hurtful, and unloving that I can hardly understand why God allows it to happen.

"Hey! Is anybody out there? Can't you see what I see? Isn't anybody listening?" I'd proclaim.

Then I realize that there are always going to be situations and tragedies that just don't, and won't, make sense to me in this life—times where justice and fairness, harmony and peace, may not be my reward for faith. Nevertheless, my hope is that, in my desire to fully embrace the Spiritual aspects of my life, I have created the ability to respond to negativity in a more peaceful and balanced way.

> ♥ Respond to negativity in a more peaceful and balanced way. ♥

I start with the vital assumption that Someone IS out there, that He is listening, and that His picture is a whole lot bigger than mine! So…I trust that, "this, too, shall pass."

The more my faith grows, the more I realize that having faith (knowing God, having Spirituality—whatever you want to call it) is not going to actually insulate me from life's problems. What it does do is balance my response to those problems, and that is a key factor in physical healing. Additionally, as my Spirituality (or my beliefs & faith) connects me to what the world might call religion, I find additional inspirational tools and recipes of hope there, as well.

♥ Knowing Over Knowledge

It seems less complicated to us when we lean on our mental abilities to think our way out of difficult situations, but I would choose my heart's "knowing" over my head's "knowledge" any time. Learning to trust faith is almost an oxymoron, isn't it? Trust is a choice each one of us has to make for ourselves. My personal relationship with the concept of a higher power (God) changes, deepens and matures as I continue to choose trust through my life's difficulties, over and over again.

That's not to say I've given up responsibility for my life, but, I believe that struggling with life's challenges, in faith, is exactly how I am to learn my life's lessons in belief. I don't think it's a cop-out to say that I let God use my pain to demonstrate His power of healing. It's something I've learned to embrace. As my faith becomes stronger, my lessons are revealed more clearly, and I believe God delights in using the things of this world to get His point across to me.

♥ Natural healing is really all about faith, you know? ♥

You may be considering acknowledging a higher power for the very first time right now; if that is so, I'm thrilled that my book could create a loving moment for your consideration; however, no matter where you are on your Spiritual pathway toward home, the key is to take the time to really experience each blessing of each pivotal moment in your life, and keep moving forward down that path.

In order to really understand natural healing and formulate a functional Self♥Love Potion, you have to be willing to accept, as truth, that there IS a power greater than yourself. I guess you'll just have to trust me on this point, but I believe with all my heart that if you ask for guidance from the knowing in your heart, your entire being—physical, mental, and emotional—will follow you wherever you are lead, and you WILL be lead. That escort is essential to balanced healing!

> ♥ Ask for guidance from the knowing in your heart…
> You will be lead. ♥

♥ Do Your Homework

Therefore, for the purposes of this book, I will refer to the knowing-higher power, as "He," "Spirit," or "God." I mean no disrespect and no slight is intended if you recognize another name. For me, these words represent expressions of articulatable thoughts. I have come to a place in my own Spiritual journey where I am comfortably at peace, calling my greater power by the names of Jesus, Spirit, and God.

Am I saying you must? No, I encourage you to seek truth for yourself. Do your homework and you will find your own language. It is certainly your choice whether or not to accept a relationship with a higher power as an intimate part of your life, and there's no shortage in this world of "Higher Powers" from which to choose.

There is an entire Spiritual smorgasbord out there! If you want the truth, you will find it, if you look deep enough. Just be sure of what's in the fruit salad before you eat the entire serving.

As a new seeker of truth through the eyes of Nature, you may see Spirituality like a giant rainbow of choices. My point is that you must have the desire to see the rainbow before you can open your eyes to the beauty of it. In some cases, even, re-open them, which can be quite difficult to do during the times of your life when it feels as if your heart has been ripped out of your very chest, and, as you're chasing after it, you smash your only pair of glasses beneath your own feet! Been there, done that, too!

♥ Inspiration

Inspiration to see is the whole purpose of my telling you my personal stories. I'm encouraging you to take the journey, and I'm simply offering you some company along the way. My desire is to encourage you to do some homework for yourself, and perhaps you'll be inspired to believe that something greater than you does exist out there. Knowing that I may be your encourager gives me the courage to speak my own truth and paint you these pictures of inspiration through the conversations I have with the inanimate objects, metaphors, facts, and fantasies of this book.

> ♥ I believe Love is God's message, and it is the inspiration for the writing of this book. ♥

I felt called to write it—not to change the world, but because truth is simply contagious, and I want to share what I've learned. Who knows, maybe you'll be the one to change the world!

I'm not real proud of some of the personal stories I'll share with you throughout this book. As a matter of fact, I'm downright embarrassed by some of my mistakes.

How is it possible that my past can look like that when, all this time, I thought I was doing the right thing? I hear myself say as I read these pages.

I had some extraordinarily poor misconceptions about love as a youth! However, I've kept my faith through it all. It's that faith that leads me to believe that if I have the courage to share my blunders with you, perhaps they can be used for good in your life and serve a purpose after all. Perhaps they will even give you the courage to trust in your own life again, as well. Maybe they will make you laugh and smile, even if it's just for a moment. However they are received, I believe God can use our time together to create something beautiful for us both. Finding your bliss from Self♥Love is a choice, just as love is still a daily choice for me, even now.

♥ Strong Enough to Begin

If you aren't currently based in a relationship that gives you permission to take a loving moment for your mistakes along the way, then let me be that permission-giver now. Let me provide you with some alternative routes to buoyancy, when you feel like a rock is hanging from a rope around your neck. That's what my friends did for me, and it made all the difference in the world.

♥When getting your needs met feels like a matter of life and death, you tend to take whatever life offers! ♥

Yet, once you're strong enough to begin to learn your own lessons and create your own recipes, you will enjoy doing it! Self♥Love may require you to let go of the hands you were once anxiously holding on to in the beginning, and inspire you to start trying some things on your own. It may even feel like you are rejecting some of the people you once desperately relied on daily. But the truth is, when you begin to understand how God wants to work in your life, Self♥Love may require you to reject some of the actions offered by some of those helping hands. You don't necessarily have to reject the person that hand is attached to, although to them it may seem like it, but you know what? Do it anyway. Self♥Love demands truth, and as you grow, you will see the truth of your friendships clearly.

♥It's okay; you're still going to be okay. ♥

Gently let go of the past and move on to the future in a loving way. Be patient with yourself and others and offer your Self♥Love recipes to those around you as you discover what works best for you. Remember, good friends will always be there for you, no matter how many times you get the recipes wrong!

I hope you will laugh at my mistakes as I offer you some validation to grieve and make mistakes of your own. Once you get the lessons, you can begin to produce your own personally empowering Self♥Love recipe, or several of them, if you like.

♥The Following Chapters

In the following chapters, I invite you to take a walk with me through Nature's four seasons. You can catalogue your own experiences in part two of this book, marked "Self♥Love Recipe Cards." The catch is, you must decipher each of Nature's messages according to the quality of your own life's lessons. In other words, it's going to take some personal "moments" to extract the individual ingredients you will need to create your own potions.

We will begin our journey by taking a brief look at life through Nature's Eyes. Unfortunately, it was a broken heart that helped me find Nature's recipes of Self♥Love, so in these first few pages I am going to give you a peek at my own self-loathing.

But please, don't get distracted by my personal saga! This book is not about a broken heart; it's really a story about faith, authentic love, patience, hope, and healing in the most unexpected moments of life. Just keep reading. By the end of the book, you will have traveled through some exciting and imaginative imagery that, I hope, will enlighten you and make you smile! Each chapter will begin with a Loving Word followed by a Small Tale that will set the flavor for each season's chapter. It is my wish that you will enjoy the journey and share it with others.

> ♥This book is not about a broken heart♥ It's really a story about authentic love and hope! ♥

♥Re-acquainting Myself with Nature

♥When I first began experimenting with the formulations for my Self♥Love Potions, I spent a lot of time re-acquainting myself with Nature and her cycles. Most of my Self♥Healing formulas come from trial and error and countless hours of cleaning up major disasters.

I learned how the seasonal changes intimately affected my recipes. With or without my permission, as Nature comes and goes my chemistry and energy move along with her. Eventually, I began writing down some of the directions Nature was pulling me in, and thus began my first Self♥Love recipe folder. After demolishing enough of my favorite cooking pans and kitchen towels, I learned to pay closer attention to Nature's guidance.

> ♥Don't mix the wrong ingredients…at the wrong time.♥

♥ Five Distinct Directions ♥

I found that there were five distinct directions Nature moves in:

- ♥ Physical
- ♥ Mental
- ♥ Emotional
- ♥ Spiritual
- ♥ Social

As well, there are four seasons in which she shifts:

- ♥ Fall
- ♥ Winter
- ♥ Summer
- ♥ Spring

Dr. Fred Schofield, a terrific chiropractor and mentoring friend of mine, once told me, "*The more you know, the more you know you don't know.*" And here is where that statement starts to make perfect sense.

♥ The Mind

Take the direction of the mind, for instance. Too much thinking can send you down the mental pathway of living a lifestyle of a control-freak. Ever met someone like that? They generally have a question for everything and in some cases, never come to a conclusion on anything while having an answer for everything. At the opposite end of the mental spectrum is the person who does not spend enough time thinking which can lead to challenges in their lifestyle of poor discernment, lack of judgment, or inability to choose all together. You see, balance in the mental realm is very important because to much or too little thinking can lead to the same loss of ability to choose, and that my friend is our greatest gift; Free will and the ability to use it wisely. Want to know what I have found to be the buffering and balancing agent for the mind? Yup, you guessed it...belief.

See, I believe that there is a big difference between the knowledge of the mind and knowing in the heart. I believe that it is the heart that holds the key to the knowing of all the fundamental ingredients necessary to produce a perfect potion.

> ♥ Peace of mind can come from the process of investigation. ♥

Peace of mind can come from the process of investigation, and the decision to form an opinion about issues for which we may not truly have all the definitive answers. It is what we choose to believe that turns us on to knowing. That knowing may be based in part on knowledge which has converted our thoughts into feelings of belief, or it may come about simply because the mind has exhausted all other possibilities of explanation. Either way, knowing and knowledge are not one in the same thing, yet they are dependent upon one another to exist.

> ♥ Okay, take a deep breath and re-read that paragraph...(smile) ♥

Basically, all I am saying is that belief can become a very powerful ingredient in the Self♥Love Potion-making process, regardless of whether you start in your head, or in your heart. As a matter of fact, it's Self♥Love Potion ingredient number one!

Ok, here's how this works: In the back of this book under "Self♥Love Potion Recipe Cards" you will find all of the ingredients' worksheets. You can go directly to the exercise when prompted throughout the following chapters of this book, or you may choose to continue reading the stories and begin your potions at a later time. It's completely up to you. A side note however: if you choose to do the exercises later on, don't procrastinate so long that you never get them done. It makes for a messy kitchen. ♥

So, let's get busy with our first recipe, shall we! Turn to the self help work book section, and complete the following ingredient worksheet.

 # Self♥Love Potion Ingredients

#1 ♥*Spirituality. Your personal connection to a higher power.*

♥What about Physical, Emotional, and Social Realms?

Now that we have discussed the Spiritual and, briefly, the mental aspects of healing, you may be asking yourself, "What about physical, emotional, and social?" Right! Sure, we need well-balanced recipes for all five areas of our lives.

> ♥ Yes, it does help to like what you see in the mirror. ♥

Of course it helps our Self♥Love Potions if we like what we see in the mirror, so physical, chemical, and nutritional health recipes are needed. I've added some great beginning recipes in the workbook section of this book, under "Seasonal Nutrition."

♥ Emotional

In the emotional realm, ♥ moments can take on an entire life of their own. They can lead your heart closer toward the truth, or harden your heart and lead you though a maze of "busy avoidance trails."

There is an existing influence in the emotional realm that can be a particularly volatile ingredient, if not stabilized while adding it to your potions. Certainly emotional imbalances can be caused by chemical, mental, and even social situations, but again I refer to the concept of belief to help stabilize an emotion.

A great deal of emotional stability comes from hope; sometimes, hope comes with the learning of the lessons, which grows faith, which then strengthens your belief, and so on.

Learning an emotional lesson isn't always easy, either. It may require you to go "through" some pain, as opposed to avoiding it!

> ♥ You can't get to the next lesson until you go through the first one. ♥

"You can't get to the next lesson until you go through the first one," my Grammy used to tell me.

On my own journey, there was a point when I discovered that I couldn't sit still long enough to even know I was emotionally hurting. That just made matters worse for me. It was a very difficult emotional lesson for me to learn when I found out that if I couldn't stand to be alone with me, there weren't going to be whole lot of other people in this world who were going to want to be alone with me, either. Once I was willing to slow down, go through, and come to terms with some pretty painful emotions, I eventually balanced out my emotional and social directions.

♥ Social

This brings us to the social direction. This realm of the body is basically, the actions you take in the world with everything your head and heart learns in life. Moving gracefully about in this world is a key aspect in keeping your Self♥Love Potions from turning rancid once you've perfected a recipe—especially if you want to share that recipe with others.

Hopefully, my words will be graceful in leading you through the pages of this book. My goal is to "fellowship" with you. Yeah, soak up some of your social time. But time spent alone with you might not be such a bad thing after all.

> ♥ Formulate your own recipes and share them with the rest of the world! ♥

Everyone's taste buds are different, but I'll bet you're capable of developing a blue ribbon-winning social formula from the ingredients right in your own kitchen! So here we go, let's travel through the seasons and see what we have in common, shall we!

Chapter Two

Chapter Two~

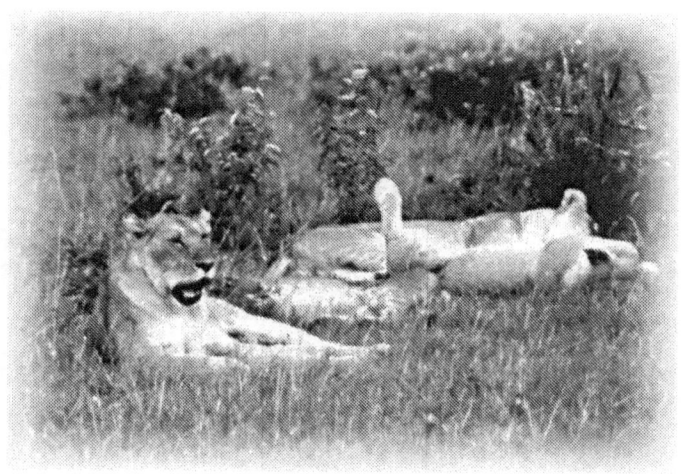

♥A Loving Voice

You are good enough to live and love, as the Spirit intended; just as you are, just as God made you, and surely will lead you…Through Nature's Eyes.

~Seasons

To the casual observer, the prairie may appear to be devoid of life. Smoldering rocks and charcoal's ash cover the hillside that was once full of Nature's color.

The howling sound of the westward winds blow seeds from across the riverbank, as Nature provides for her seemingly lifeless plain.

But there, in the distance, in the direction of the sunset, just beyond the lazily dropping temperature, there is movement. A patch of green brush remains. Only the tips of the shrub have browned; the base is lush, green, and full— a color that can only be pulled from the mineral rich soil of naturally charred earth.

Under the shrub's shaded offering lie the lioness and her cub. Unhurried and seemingly indifferent to the changing season, steadily moving about the grounds, the lioness rolls to her back, extending her left hind leg to the heavens as she gracefully inspects her front paw.

Stretching and yawning, she rolls to her side, where she can keep a watchful eye on her energetic young cub, whose black nose is dug deep into the ashy soil for its play.

With hind legs bent, back arched and ears pointed, the cub delights in a deliberate attack upon the floating embers.

Yes, to the casual observer, the land may look injured and devoid of life, but through the eyes of Nature we are offered a tender view of the shifting "moments" in which life is continued and order restored—a view of Nature's seasons .~C

♥Through Nature's Eyes

♥There is a perfect harmony to be witnessed through the spectacular phenomena of Nature's colors and her changing seasons. We can use Nature's eyes to see life, if our own have been closed.

As soon as I opened my eyes to Nature, there, in the presence of mist and light, several different colors came in to view, and, with them, the desire to "take a moment" to feel the energy and vibration that accompanies Nature's messages!

Nature has so many voices, so many physically occurring energy cycles that are taking place, right now:

- ♥Darkness to sunlight
- ♥Full moons to new moons
- ♥Hormones and metabolism
- ♥Menstruation and menopause
- ♥Sleep, dream, and waking states
- ♥Instincts, growth, and aging

And that's to name only a few. Then there are all kinds of colorful vibrations, and they affect these cycles as well.

There is:

♥ music,   ♥ sight,
♥ sound,   ♥ touch,
♥ taste,   ♥ smell; and
♥ hearing.

Just as the changing seasons restore order and supply energy and harmony to the earth, nature's energy cycles are available to restore, energize, and harmonize our lives. Nowhere else but in nature can we see the awesome power of God so beautifully displayed for our appreciation and contemplation.

♥ A Rainbow

Did you know that if you were to combine all of the beautiful colors of a rainbow in equal proportions you would end up with only one color?

> ♥ Yup, pure light! I call it Truth. ♥

Do you know what the opposite of pure light is? Darkness. See, if Nature were to combine all her colors in an unfaithful or disorganized fashion, the result would be mass chaos and darkness. No love, no hate—just nothingness. I'll bet you didn't know that a rainbow couldn't be seen in the presence of even ordinary darkness. Really! Thank God, Nature does not make those mistakes.

Through nature, God has put into place a very specific and wonderful array of colors, sights, sounds, foods, and vibrations.

> ♥These vibrations allow us an unrivaled way in which to connect to everlasting healing, and to God.♥

♥Deep & Progressive

I've learned to relish the secrets revealed by paying close attention to this deep, progressive body of energy. I have take many a "moment" with Nature. When I view the seasons through the loving Spirit I believe created them, I embrace, in childlike wonder, the excitement each new season of my life brings.

I get to enjoy these deep and intimate connections with an authority that has a design and purpose for my very life, but only when I take the moments to look for them. I just have to remember to get beyond that left-brained or casual observer's perspective in order to see my life through the loving eyes of Nature.

♥A Birthday Moment

During one tumultuous birthday moment I asked myself if I could in fact stop Nature somehow? You know, stay young forever, and be bliss-fully happy right where I was. Could I really avoid the lessons? The reply came deep from within.

Do you really want to stop the lessons? And, if you could make time stand still, you don't really want to suspend the future joys of your life by staying where you are now, do you?

I suppose I would be happy just slowing the lessons from time to time, but even if I could interfere with the processes of Nature, the truth is, "… ♥Nature always has, always will, find a way around my road roadblocks!" ♥

Nature's cycles straightforwardly come and go, with or without my permission. But by spending intimate moments with Nature, I've learned to tap into her cycles and use her wisdom as a door through which I can invite beauty beyond years to my life.

I remember my mom forever telling me, "Beauty comes from the inside first." Self♥Love was what she was really talking about. Through seeking out moments, and being willing to keep moving forward as I held Nature's hand,

♥ I've learned to awaken to the strength and inspiration Nature is extending to me through her predictable and powerful cycles. ♥

♥ The Truth of Who We Are

♥ In the Midwest, the seasons are far more distinguishable than sunny Southern California, where I live. Nevertheless, we get a new energy cycle, commonly referred to as a season, approximately every three months.

During each one of Nature's seasons—Winter, Spring, Summer, and Fall—Nature will offer up four basic formulas to aid you in the production of your Self♥Love recipes.

♥ Winter is resting.
♥ Spring is building.
♥ Summer is expending.
♥ Fall is cleansing.

Now, granted, Nature's view is much more glamorous than mine, but before we dive in to the seasons, let's start with knowing the truth of who we are, so that we are able to accept responsibility for our actions before we leave the past behind us.

> ♥Knowing the truth of who we are will help us accept responsibility for our past and future actions.♥

♥Knowing the truth of who you are is about learning, and then accepting, your strengths and weaknesses. Stepping out into truth's light requires courage, but is necessary in order to move forward in peace. Sometimes that reflection of truth, well, (Yikes!); It's not always pretty!

> ♥The truth is…I've always found it easier to look at someone else, before I looked at myself.♥

But, eventually, I'd find the courage—the right recipe, the coping skills, whatever—to deal with my life's weaknesses and issues constructively. That would enable me to then move forward in truth. There is a wide range of feelings that accompanied the truth of my own self-loathing. Yet, there is a gentle strength to be uncovered through the greatest heartbreaks and challenges of life, and my Spirit delights in my choices to discover them. As a matter of fact, that brings us to Self♥Love Potion ingredient number two. It's time for you to find this truthful ingredient and add it to your own potion.

 # Self♥Love Potion Ingredients

#1 ♥Spirituality. Your personal connection to a higher power.
#2 ♥Knowing your truths and accepting responsibility.

My Broken Pieces

♥In these next few pages I offer you the stories of my personal brokenness, weaknesses, poor choices, and heartbreaks. Now, I realize that many of your struggles may be far worse than any of my most excruciating days, so I am not offering up my misfortunes to engage your pity. I offer up the tenderest parts of my life, honestly and sincerely, to encourage you to persevere through your own struggles, no matter how painful they may feel in the moment. My desire is to encourage you to look for, and find, the little hidden gems of healing lessons within each mishap of your life, and to use those gems to help others heal in return. It's simple really, but the results can be dramatic!

♥ The Early Years ♥

I'll not bore you with the complete details of my youth, but all I ever wanted was to be and feel loved. My mom had it tough trying to raise us three kids after my dad died, and she did one heck of a job. But one thing led to another, and I ended up leaving home with disillusionment, just as my brothers before and after me. Those early years of lost love affected each of us differently.

Psychologists believe that strong attachments develop when our emotional and physical needs are met, or not met, and that they begin with the parent-infant bond.

> ♥ We often re-enact the original bonding experiences we felt as a child with the people we Fall for as adults. ♥

I suppose losing my dad at the age of seven could have had something to do with the romantic notion that a "Mr. Right" was my missing piece. Or maybe it was all those darn Cinderella stories that did it to me. But regardless of why, the fact is that I thought the right guy would fill all my voids, and that happiness could only mean a husband who would love me forever.

So, I left home with nothing but the clothes on my back, and set off into the romantic sunset. I had already met the man of my dreams while taking night courses at junior college, during my last year in high school, but I ended up running away and moving in with the parents of a boy I had met earlier that Summer. I was little more than nineteen.

This nice young man's parents offered me a room and food while I continued my college education and dated their son. To help pay the expenses, I worked part-time as a medical assistant, and as long as I was a full-time student I received money from my deceased father's social security fund. I've always felt a little guilty about taking that check away from my mom's budget though. Sorry, Mom. (Smile).

♥The Man of My Dreams

So, back to the reason for telling you this story—back to the man of my dreams. Well, obviously my "Mister Right" was not the boy I was dating…he was a young, partying, fun-boy with big, muscular arms and a smile that could light up a room. He was everything but ready to settle down when we met, but we fast became the best of friends. There were pains in my young abdomen at the time we met, and they were getting worse. The doctor I was working for told me he didn't think I would ever be able to have children. He said it was looking like I was heading for surgery and soon!

♥Oh, no! I wanted kids! ♥

At the tender age of nineteen, I found my biological clock was already counting down. Of course, instead of relying on God's will for my life (not that I could have even followed it clearly back then, anyway), I took matters into my own hands.

Since having a child out of wedlock was out of the question, and my partying Mr. Right was not ready to settle down, I decided to marry Mr. Right-Now: Yes, the boy whose parents I was living with. Off I went into that logically romantic sunset, without my sunglasses on!

Yes, I rushed into that marriage alright. But from today's perspective, it does not matter to me whether I made the wrong choice for the right reason or vice versa. Within a year after having a little baby girl, I did end up having a complete hysterectomy. So that marriage provided me with a very special glimpse of heaven that I see reflected in the face of my daughter every day since I made that choice. Today, I know so much more about psychosomatic and metaphysical causation that, had I known back then what I know now, I may have been able to prevent an agonizing surgery. Nonetheless, I am blessed with the knowing of the joy of childbirth, and I am at peace with the choice I made to leap into that marriage.

But back to the story of this woman's misconceptions about love. It only begins here.

> ♥ It doesn't matter if it was the wrong choice for the right reason, or the other way around, today I am blessed and at peace with it. ♥

Although I felt blessed at the time of my daughter's birth, my heart still felt empty and I silently longed for love. It was easy for me to provide for others what I considered love to be, but why couldn't I feel it myself?

"Mr. Right" had remained my best friend through all the major events of my life and in retrospect , that was a really poor choice for my marriage. (I share that gem with you now, But you know what they say, hind sight is 20/20.) Anyway, he was there for my wedding, the birth of my daughter, my surgeries, and gradually it became clear that what we were sharing was more than just friendship. I felt as if he were offering me the very thing I wanted most in my life: love, real love. I really believed he was my soul mate, my one and only Mr. Right, my single chance at real love. He was finally ready for a girl like me. The problem was, I belonged to someone else.

My husband acknowledged the look in my eyes when he listened to me talk about my best friend or watched us together, laughing and acting silly. He could tell, though I never spoke the words, he could no longer deny the truth of the circumstances. Being the wonderful man that he was, he made it easy for me to follow my heart. In retrospect, he made it perhaps too easy, but nonetheless, we ended up parting as friends, and though the journey was painful for him at times, we still remain friends to this day.

Now available to love's promise, I was eager to find love and happiness within the loving embrace of the man whom I thought was my Mr. Right. I wanted to have a 50th wedding anniversary, sip lemonade while swaying in a rocking chair on the front porch of our home, and watch our grandkids play in our front yard with this man. I believed we would look back over our life together and feel lucky to have had the chance at living an existence in genuine love together. Obviously, I never gave myself a chance to feel, pray, or think…I just rode off into another sunset. Only this time I was sure it would lead to that fairytale finale.

♥ Real Love?

Together my new husband and I created loving dreams of a future. I worked for an urgent care center, and he provided the loving and nurturing support of a father-figure for my daughter as he pursued a chiropractic education. My daughter was going to have the love and home life I never knew. This is the way I'd always dreamed it would be!

Our wedding day was the most beautiful day of my life, besides the birth of my daughter. In this man's arms I anticipated achieving the feeling of real love once and for all. The love I felt for my daughter was the most profound feeling of love I had ever experienced, yet I still believed the missing piece I was searching for rested within the promise of living my life with this man. I existed to complement and support my husband's every vision for our lives. I adopted his dreams as my own.

> ♥This man had become my everything, and there wasn't much room for anything else. ♥

There was nothing I wouldn't have given or done for this man. I even changed my profession to earn experience in the chiropractic field so I could create the office of his dreams after he graduated. My desire was to give him the very best of everything I had to offer, and if I didn't have it, I would find it for him.

Years later, we had finished building the second of our two chiropractic practices. Oh, the hours spent marketing and painting walls! It was amazing to see how far I had traveled, for love's sake.

> ♥I kept thinking that if I just worked hard enough and long enough, eventually I would feel the love. ♥

I tried everything I could think of to find that harmony I had prayed for all my life. By the sixth year of our marriage, I had already begun experimenting with Self♥Love Potions, trying all kinds of different recipes: acting, gymnastics, politics. I guess I knew something was wrong, but my conscious mind just hadn't figured it out yet.

I began going within, on a deeper Spiritual journey. I could feel God nudging me, stronger than ever before. Understanding what it took to be a Godly wife became my focus. That drive continued to grow until, eventually, I found myself completing the last of the three-year process that it took to prove myself worthy of a church blessing on our already nine-year-old marriage. We renewed our wedding vows in the early morning hours of a beautiful Spring day in April. This would be the last April we would spend together as husband and wife.

♥ The Final Year ♥

Six months later, October, would mark the month that the final adoption papers for my daughter were to be officially signed. Over those previous nine years, my daughter's biological father hadn't come around much. I can't say I blame the poor guy, though. Our friends all had assumed my husband was my daughter's father, and in some cases we manufactured stories to perpetuate that belief. I suppose we thought we were doing the right thing at the time. My daughter knew who her biological father was, and though I encouraged her to maintain a relationship with him, I could tell it was uncomfortable for my husband, so I never pushed the issue. Today, however, through a cycle of providential events, my daughter has a positive relationship with her biological father, as well as her stepfather. See, God can use anything for good if we simply let Him, but that's another story.

Anyway, back to the tale. To the outside world, we were the perfect little family. Two new cars in the garage, a beautiful new house in an affluent neighborhood, my daughter attending a private school, a successful business. I had gotten the church's approval and renewed my wedding vows, and the final missing piece that would pull the whole picture together that final year was my husband's decision to legally adopt my daughter. This was going to be the year that I could start to slow down a little and enjoy the love I had built into my life, or so I thought.

Remember that mask of determination I told you I always wore? The harder things get for me, the harder I push to make things go my way. By Mid-September of that final year, my husband had already mysteriously lost two wedding rings, and I had noticed that ever since the renewal of our wedding vows, five months earlier, he had been acting distant and mysterious, more than usual. Something was up; I just did-n't know what. So, I pushed on.

It was only a month before the signing of those adoption papers, and my husband and I were headed off to Hawaii for an herb convention and a kind of second honeymoon. While on the islands, I offered to buy another wedding ring to signify the beginning of a wonderful, fresh start for us in God's eyes! I believed that the church's recognition of our marriage meant that I had been forgiven for my past choices, and now God was really going to bless my life and my marriage. I was so excited about getting my husband a new ring to signify our love!

However, we ended up having such an argument about it that he walked off along the beach for hours by himself, obviously deep in thought. We were arguing about everything! The next day while on a paddle boat, he confessed his thoughts to me. He felt he needed some space and wanted to be on his own. "It's not you. It's me," he said.

That statement just bounced off my mask of determination to pre-serve love's promise, and I walked toward our hotel room with confi-dence. *Hah,* I thought, *He wouldn't dare! Not now; not after all we've been through together; not after all I've done for him. He just renewed his wedding vows to me only five months ago. And besides, he's going to be adopting my angel next month!*

Within the hour, he returned to our hotel room bed, demonstrating and confessing his everlasting love. But I knew something was still wrong. I could feel it in my bones. I didn't want to believe what my gut was suggesting. Was there someone else messing with my true love's promise? I shuddered at the thought.

After ten days in the Hawaiian Islands, we returned to our daily routine back in California, and I to that familiar feeling—the feeling of being unloved. My husband's behavior became more and more unpredictable. One minute he was calling me at home to check on me and tell me he loved me, and the next he was defending his absences and long hours away. He grew more and more silent and mysterious, taking long walks along the California coast after work (or so he said).

♥ Hallucinations & Accusations

Was he driving me crazy, or was I driving myself crazy? I became outwardly and verbally suspicious that the greatest threat to my heart's desire came in the form of a blond-haired patient. He told me I was crazy, but after another week of hallucinations and hurling accusations, I followed up on a gut-wrenching hunch. Finally, I caught him on the phone with "HER." It WAS the neighbor who was leaving her husband, and needed hours of counseling from mine. I stood there in the doorway with a plate of food in my hand, absorbing the final blow to an already broken heart.

October 7th, four days before he was to sign the final adoption papers, six months after renewing our wedding vows, and after years of knowing and loving this man, it was finished. No counseling, no reconciliation, no nothing; just…gone. Yes, my friends, this was, indeed, the greatest heartbreak of my life, and the greatest lesson in love, as well.

♥ Did I Already Know?

So what happened, you ask? Had he been trying to leave me for a number of years? Had he been planning this with HER for months, days, weeks? Did I already know he was gone before he really left? Was my desperate need for love so strong that I didn't want to see the truth?

Friends close to us at the time later suggested that I had been ignoring the signs for a number of years, and felt I was trying to hold it all together and cover up the truth of my brokenness through religion and Spirituality. Perhaps all of the above is true. Perhaps it was just a matter of time before I would have known the truth, anyway. Our lives were going in different directions. I was having Monday night Bible studies, and he, *Monday Night Football,* with her. I take a small amount of peace knowing that his leaving really didn't have anything to do with HER, because if it wasn't her, it would have been someone else. What it had to do with was ME! Like I said, every choice has a consequence.

One choice I am so very grateful for making was the choice to fill myself with God's word during the last few years of our marriage. Because I had made those choices before my life fell apart, it was easier to pull thorough. God remained my stability when everything else was gone.

♥ Couldn't Get Any Worse, Could It?

He was now planning a wedding with this woman who was about to have his baby, and all I knew was that I had an entire life's plan with a husband I adored one minute, and he was giving it all to someone else the next! When he left, it felt like all of my dreams for the future had left with him, and I began refocusing on the idea that maybe I was somehow unworthy of real love.

> *It wasn't supposed to be like this,* I thought. *"Is this what happens when you really love someone? Is love really supposed to hurt this bad?*

I kept asking myself the craziest of questions, such as "How come he could walk away from me with such ease, when all I could feel was helplessness, sadness, and anxiety?" Loving him defined who I was. I felt like a little child. I literally believed I needed my husband's love in order to survive. Where did I go wrong?

♥ Clueless

Although consciously I knew I wasn't literally going to die, and today I am so much more than "the one who was left," at the time it sure felt like I was going through hell, in every part of my body! I really thought

I wasn't capable of making it on my own. I was clueless. I had spent so much of my life building his life, and hiding behind a mask of strength and determination to make it all work, that I really knew very little about the truth of the fragile creature that lived underneath it all. I felt like my life was slipping away, and somehow it felt like it was all my fault. All I wanted was to be loved. *Is that so much to ask for from life?* I heard myself screaming to the heavens.

At one point, a member of my own family started to question my competence as a wife, which was the lowest point for me. When that relative chose my ex-husband's company over mine, I began to sink deeper and deeper into that familiar feeling of not being good enough, and not being loved. I vacillated between the hope Spirituality provided and the despair my mind had for the future of my life. I stood there naked with my heart in my hands. Falling to my knees,I begged God to stop the pain.

♥ Conflicting Collision of Emotions ♥

The traditions and rituals of my church prohibited me from the very communion I had sought, as the details of my broken marriage were put on display. My Spiritual shelter had become a place of mortal pain. But when my husband asked me to say it was a mutual break up, so as not to upset the "family" practice, I knew I needed professional help to deal with the emotions.

Before I found out my husband's girlfriend was pregnant with his child, I begged for reconciliation and counseling. Oh, how I humiliated myself. But I thought, that's what real love required of me. I just couldn't let go.

Have you ever seen a child clutching a baby blanket? You know what they do when you try to take it away from them, without offering something in its place? Yup, that was me: scared to death. I would have done anything.

My husband figured he had paid his counseling dues years earlier, when we had had a bad experience in counseling after a car accident. It was suggested that my husband attend a counseling session or two with me. My husband thought the counselor was full of you-know-what, but went anyway. When the counselor began attacking our relationship (yeah, I took it as an attack on me), I got up and walked out. I wasn't going to allow anyone to attack the very veins of my heart and suggest that my marriage had problems.

As a matter of fact, I ignored problems altogether. I would stand in defense of my husband's honor, denying that he would entertain a woman bearing gifts of food late in the evening in his office. And many times I would simply look the other way as he would hand out his business card to the cocktail waitress, smile, and say, "She is just going to be a patient, baby." There were ex-patients who pleaded with me to "get a clue," letters from co-workers and ex-employees who spoke of situations that I refused to believe. Will I ever really know the truth behind any of those stories? Who knows, but today I can hear these friends tell me their stories and see for myself what I was so blind to then. Oh, the hell I put myself through...all in the name of love.

♥The Authorities

I bought every book I could find on reconciling a broken marriage. One book said, be strong, change the locks, make him miss you; another said, get on your knees and beg forgiveness; one more still said this has nothing to do with your will—let God handle it.

Needless to say, I immediately sought out a qualified counselor, just to break up the monotony of the long crying jags. I'd get on my knees and pray that I could stop feeling, only to end up heaving my insides out into the toilet, praying that if I could just feel loved, everything would be okay.

Occasionally, while lying motionless after a crying spell, I would remind myself that my husband was now with this younger blonde; the one with "great athletic legs" who was now having his baby. She made a great living as a mortgage broker, and could offer him all the playmate time that he so desperately needed, as well as the toys to go with it, without all the responsibility of a nagging, religious, controlling, needy, emotionally devastated mom of a wife. If you were he, what would you have chosen? Then I heard myself whisper, "For God's sake, love; real love!"

I didn't know what to do I moved back and forth between wearing a mask of strength, and just flat out breaking down. Then I'd find the strength to start crying all over again. Somewhere along the line of my life, I had gotten it stuck up in my head that I had to have a man in my life in order to be whole. Now that my husband was gone, I felt like I was nothing at all. I could write an entire separate book on how afraid I was that this form of thinking was going to affect my daughter and make her a love freak! That's when I found the strength to discover the truth of who I really was.

♥ More Choices

Some of that counseling work was finally beginning to pay off. I learned a little about the psychology of my pain; that quite possibly I was feeling as emotionally vulnerable as the child I once was, when my life literally depended on the love of my Daddy. His death, and the withdrawal of my husband's attention, evoked those same feelings of helplessness, sadness, and lovelessness. Just as I had learned to be strong for my mom's sake after my dad died, I had picked a man who needed that kind of strength to help him open and run his business. When my focus on his business began to shift, so did our relationship.

I could have gone down one of several pathways, a hardened heart being one of them. I could have suppressed the pain in my heart, ignored it, and pretended it didn't exist. I could have lashed out. Oh, trust me, I wanted to once or twice. I still laugh, because the few times I let myself enjoy even a few minutes of unfriendly fire, "Unreasonable and irrational," he would say.

Thank God he never knew just how irrational and unreasonable I really was beneath that heavy mask of control. Fortunately, God didn't see fit to abandon me while I figured it all out. Although I rebelled against the "traditional religious acts" of my faith because I found them to be too painful to endure, I still had my beliefs, and a growing intimate relationship with God.

Eventually, I learned to be patient with me, and grew wise in contrast to the pain. I became strong by holding on to my faith and beliefs, not for his love's sake, but to keep my heart from becoming hardened and shutting down altogether.

♥The Lesson

In the beginning of these lessons I had to learn the truth. Now remember, my husband was the doughnut glaze over the "believing that I was not worthy of being loved" lesson, so the lessons that followed him leaving me all had a recognizable flavor to them.

Learning to give up the pursuit of romantic love in order to recognize the deep healing properties that Spiritual Self♥Love can provide was a choice I had to make, one day at a time. As time went on, the lesson became clear, and new lessons were able to take their turns.

I began to emerge from issue-to-issue living, to life's existence in between the issues. That's where I found life's moments and the recipes that are now working in my life. There were many times those moments weren't easy to experience, even if I do make light of them in some of my stories, now.

I've had to work through a wide range of emotions—shock, rage, sadness, frustration, disillusionment, resentment, and on and on—to get where I am today, and I'm still learning.

> ♥ I was struggling for so long to *be* loved that I never gave myself the time to feel the profoundness of being *unloved.* ♥

Finally, by keeping hold of God's hand through it all, I was able to let go of an unhealthy need for love, and found the desire to make some difficult changes in my perception of it altogether. As I learned my lessons, my fragile and lonely heart continued to make a number of blunders, which I will share with you later.

♥ A Little Smug?

Today, when someone tells me I sound a little smug, or like a princess sitting atop my parochial Christian soapbox, I remember all the choices I've had to make to survive some of life's most difficult moments. I'm not saying I no longer want to have the romantic love I prayed for, and you're not going to hear me complain if God's plan for me does include a big sparkly for my left hand; but, what I am saying is that I've learned, and am still learning, to replace my brokenness with the unconditional love of God, while tending to my own Self♥Love recipes as well.

By taking the time to deal with the truths of my life, the "desperate need" for romantic love has been replaced with the ability to show up in this world as a whole person, rather than the me who was constantly dashing off here and there, running from the truth of my life.

> ♥The person I dreaded being yesterday has blossomed into the person I'm happy to be today. ♥

There is pure strength in knowing, "Yes, God does love me just the way I am, but He loves me too much to leave me this way!" He's not done with me yet!

♥ Control it! ♥

In order for me to fix the things I didn't know were even broken, I had to take the ♥ moments it required to discover the weaknesses that were masquerading as strengths within me. I believed that as long as I could control it, I could keep it from hurting me. WRONG! I found out that we can't control other people! The more I tried to control what God already had planned for me, the longer it took for the lessons to even make sense to me, no matter how much faith I had.

In the beginning, the lessons just kept getting lost on me, as I kept trying to force my way through life. Every night I prayed that God would hear my prayers. Every morning I awoke looking for His answers. But every time He tried to point me in a direction I didn't want to go, I'd rebel and shout "NO, that's not the answer I was looking for!" I suppose that's when God decided to take matters into His own hands. Yup, I guess He figured He'd better do something before I destroyed our relationship altogether. And that's when I met Him face to face. No, not just another man, the Limo Driver…

♥ The Limo Driver

♥ It was from the back seat of a big black limo that I wrote most of the pages to this book. Being a control freak may have made the journey more interesting, but it sure didn't make it any easier on me, let me tell you. I was so uncomfortable with the idea of someone else navigating the rocky roads for me. Ever heard the term "back seat driver?" That was me. Constantly fighting God for control. What I needed to do was just shut my mouth for a while, just sit in the back seat of that big old Mercedes limo God was driving me around in, and get to know myself a bit.

During the bumpiest parts of the ride, when I was the most scared of finding out who I really was, I'd find the exit doors to the car locked. I'd frantically push and pull against the locked door, kicking, screaming, and yelling at the darn exits to open up.

> ♥Sometimes jumping out of the window of a moving vehicle actually made perfect sense to me, in my moments of despair. ♥

You'd think God would have been concerned about me destroying His car during these little temper tantrums I would throw, but He made it clear that He didn't want me jumping out of my life's plan completely just because the going got rough. He had locked those doors for my own protection. I get it now; but every time He did it to me then, I'd get so angry at Him!

> ♥ It doesn't much matter to Him during those "critical" navigational periods, whether He gets you there kicking and screaming behind a locked door, or just sitting there, painting your toenails. ♥

There are certain places God has to get us in our lives, and all He is concerned with during a crisis is getting you there. He'd just roll up the soundproof partition screen between us so He could focus on the rocky road ahead. I'd see Him looking back in His rearview mirror from time to time, though, and I could tell He was concerned about me hurting myself. He seemed so sure of Himself and determined, whenever I caught a glimpse of His sparkling eyes. In the end, I realized He wasn't going to let me jump out of my life's plan that easily, so I eventually learned to just sit there and paint my toenails and pout.

Pouting had always worked for me before, but it didn't seem to go over too well with God. I'd get so mad at Him because I didn't think He was listening to a word I was saying when that darn partition was up. Then, when the partition was down, I was so irritated I didn't know what to say, so I'd just sit there with my arms crossed over my chest, and complain under my breath. Little did I know that He could hear every word I was saying and thinking. Seems the entire limo was wired with this really sensitive intercom system that let Him hear the very thoughts in my head. Fortunately for me, the sound system also conveyed the true nature of my heart.

I sure am glad He knew the origin of my pain and frustrations, because I was feeling pretty bad about some of the things I had been thinking. But God never said a word to me about the anger. He always focused on my heart. That was just His way. Something about Grace, I think. My knowing that He knew was good enough for Him.

Oh, the lessons! I didn't always like them, either. Rolling down the window as we'd cruise past these fun-looking groups of people, I'd be wondering why I was stuck in the back seat of this limo. How come I had to sit here and watch all this stuff just pass my life by? How come I wasn't out there like one of those people? Surely that's who I was supposed to be. At least, that's how I saw myself. They looked like they were having all the fun, and it didn't look like they were paying any consequences for their actions, either! How come I had to?

The learning of this lesson, however, turned out to be a point in finding the true nature of my heart, beneath the anger and pain. What I found there was envy, and letting go of it was a difficult lesson to learn but an essential ingredient to my Self♥Love Potion. That's Self♥Love Potion ingredient number three. Let's stop and do that one now!

 **Self♥Love Potion Ingredients**

#1 ♥ *Spirituality. Your personal connection to a higher power.*
#2 ♥ *Knowing your Truths and accepting responsibility.*
#3 ♥ *Letting go of envy.*

♥A Means of Being Happy

The moments I spent driving past all those fun-looking people showed me that I have been provided with a means of being happy, no matter what my circumstances might be at the time.

> ♥After having enough things pass me by, I got tired of pouting—you know, being the victim. ♥

Have you ever found it easy to cry for those who are crying? I have. It's human instinct to feel bad for someone's bad luck, I think. But it was when I realized I was sad about the people that were happy that I saw myself as a jealous person. Yeah—jealous!

So, I decided to try something different. I tried rejoicing for those I saw rejoicing. And what happened was that I actually started to feel good about seeing other people who were feeling good about their own personal choices!

I learned I could always find something to be happy about, even if it wasn't about me! Does that mean I quit thinking I was the center of the universe? I don't think so…but this new way of thinking was far better than sitting there, pouting about a process for which I had asked.

There I was, sitting there pouting because someone else appeared to be enjoying something I wanted, or felt I deserved, which God wasn't giving it to me. But, since I chose to take that limo ride in the first place, it was actually my choice to be kept away from those things! Oh, how frustrating that was, until I learned a little more about the word "appear."

> ♥Things are not always what they *appear* to be. ♥

God would always say that to me with a smirk.

So anyway, there I was, safe and sound in a warm and cozy limo, with seemingly unlimited gas mileage and self-service hot beverages, and I'm complaining about wanting to be one of those people that are out there dancing in the pouring rain.

I'll bet ya, even if I had been allowed to get out there and dance, I probably would have found something else to complain about, like not having a partner to dance with, or whatever. But as I sat there, restricted in the back seat of that limo, I was aware of the pleasure that watching those people brought me. I began to tap into their excitement for life; and as I watched them, out there, dancing in joy for the choices they had made for their lives, I began to feel good myself.

> ♥I began to embrace their pleasure as my own.♥

I even smiled back at them from time to time as I sat there, listening to some cool tunes from a killer sound system in the back of my big plush limo. I realized I had it pretty good, after all. I even danced around in the back of that limo by myself a few times, and that's when I noticed out of the corner of my eye, some of those people looking at me with the same expression of envy I had for them. Perspective is a funny thing, isn't it?

> ♥Simply and Positively Protected!♥

♥In the Dark

Many of the times when I thought I was being punished, or missing out in life, I was really being protected. That's why the back seat windows of that limo had been tinted. At first I felt like God was try-ing to keep me in the dark or something. What He was really doing by providing me with those tinted windows was trying to keep the light of truth (which was so bright in contrast to my way of thinking) from blinding me altogether. In my darkest moments, I discovered some of my most empowering Self♥Love Potion recipes, and I really began to appreciate those tinted windows after a while.

It was a tough lesson for me, but when I got it, I GOT IT! God would just smile at me from the rearview mirror when He'd see the lights go on in my head, and toss me back a new color of nail polish. Then He'd wink at me as if to say, *Ready to go?* and we'd speed right back up again, off to another adventure or lesson. In some ways, I think those windows served a dual purpose, protecting me from the outside, and protecting the outside from me!

♥This Ride Will Be Continued...♥

Chapter Three

Chapter Three

♥His Vision of Her
♥Emotional Treasures of a Fall
♥Self♥Love Potions 4 & 5

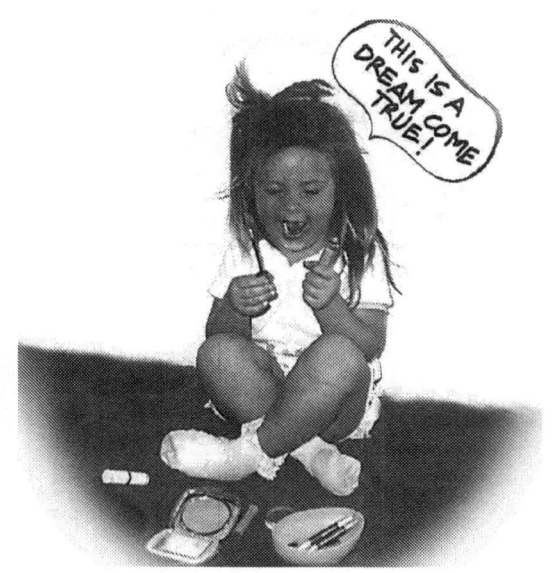

♥*A Loving Voice*

The flash and glitz may be gone, but our hearts seem to want to get beyond that anyway. Now is as good a time as any.

♥His Vision of Her

It is not the tilted head as she laughs that instills love's admiration. The crystalline tinkle in her mirth as her eyes sparkle with life's passion. It is just so, and those who love her shrug their shoulders and accept it.

We have been amused to point out her embarrassments, her predicaments; but her intent was to drink love, live life with pure appreciation.

Her moment in the sun, she'll dance in the moonlight, oft as not desiring to peel away clothing at the impulsive inspirations to feel the coolness of a mountain stream or lake.

She is all that most men dream. Spirit ablaze for the deep kiss that leaves one breathless, a child in her insecurities pouting her willful ways, then questioning if she is being unfair to her tormentors.

She is adorable, adorned with childish innocence and doubts. She exemplifies the mystical in woman. She is seductive, sensual, and alluring. She reminds a man why he seeks her gender.

Bright and dangerous in her lightning observations, she inspires the artist and challenges the cleric. She is irreverent not for scandal's sake, though she'd relish the attention, but for the righteousness born in her very being. She is a warrior for her Clan, a tigresses in defenses for her loves.

She seeks enlightenment and harmony yet is an agent for change. Adventure is her kinsmen, *but hearth and home embodies her celebration...~Wordman*

♥Emotional Treasures of a Fall

♥Although Fall officially starts September 21st, for me it starts with that little orange and yellow triangle shaped candy. As soon as I see the stores stocking their shelves with those precious little goodies, I know that I am in for a kaleidoscope of emotions and feelings that need to be processed and eliminated, to make room for a peaceful resting through the Winter cycle, which will follow next.

I just love the Fall colors: golds, oranges, browns, and yellows. These are all of Nature's cleansing colors. By eating the colors of the seasons you will be right in line with what Nature has planned for your body, as well as your heart.

Color-coding my recipe cards allows me to easily identify the season I'm working on, and keep in mind how Nature is going to lend me a hand. Interestingly enough, I have found that the dis-ease or dis-harmony in my life during Fall is quite simply Nature's way of attempting to "clean out" and restore order to it. Since Nature brings in a new energy with each season, her subtle changes in colors give me a chance to exchange crayons and prepare for what is to come next.

♥Cleaning Up the Ambiguous

I see the Fall part of a relationship as a time when I am more likely to have a heart to heart talk about what does and doesn't feel good to me. You know, clean up the ambiguous feelings, and make room for the New Year.

I find the Fall subject matter generally contains issues regarding:

♥ commitment   ♥ dedication
♥ loyalty   ♥ promise
♥ boundaries   ♥ conclusions
♥ finalization   ♥ terminations, and ♥ moving on.

It takes a lot of work to cleanse, physically, mentally, or emotionally. But Nature is so good with her timing. Winter, which is only three months away, is designed for the very things we will need most: rest and relaxation. During the Fall, however, Nature is hard at work, blowing those fruits from the trees. She doesn't much care if it's a good apple or a bad one. If you don't pick it by the end of the Fall season, she's going to move in and blow it down so the tree can rest in the Winter months ahead.

> ♥ You work hard picking the good ones,
> and let Nature do the rest. ♥

After having enough Fall recipes explode in my kitchen during the conversations I was ill-prepared for, I learned to be more organized. Nature has taught me to prepare for those Fall communications rather than just letting them happen to me.

♥The Best and Worst♥

For me, the best and worst of times of my life collide with each other during the Fall season. I go through pretty much the same routine every year.

As a youth, I anticipated with much excitement the day of my birth, which now arrives right on schedule in the month of September, year after year...after year.

However, as I've learned to confront the telltale signs of maturity, through Nature's eyes instead of my own, I release the disheartened broken image I've created in the mirror, and genuinely embrace the wisdom and purpose that age reveals. In other words, I choose to believe that Nature's graceful display of laugh lines about my face somehow illuminates the pleasures of my youth for all to see. (Smile) Nonetheless, I still begin the month of October with a mouth full of orange and yellow triangle-shaped candy corns.

♥A Final Cleansing Talk♥

It was in the second month of the Fall cleansing season (October) that the love of my life had his final Fall cleansing talk with me, leaving me with more than a decade of November memories, organic turkeys, and pumpkin pies, all of which were baked in one of the three ovens that lined my magnificent kitchen. Then one day, almost suddenly, these terrific Fall experiences were replaced with a spaghetti dinner, shared in exhaustion with my daughter, in the empty living room of a newly-painted apartment.

As I resisted the changes that were taking place in the Fall of my life at the time, I could feel myself growing weak and becoming physically ill.

> ♥No part of the body, or even one cell in the body, can be separated from the Spirit. ♥

♥The Greatest Emotional Treasures of this Particular Fall, Revealed ♥

Remember when I told you how I had spent the better part of the last few years of my marriage trying to find my confidence, and doing some in-house emotional cleansing? Only, I hadn't understood how to go about it gently just yet. I had taken up a fairly rigorous form of self-improvement. Since I internally knew something was not right in my marriage, but couldn't put my finger on it, I began praying and committing myself to learning whatever was required of me to become what I perceived as a more loving wife.

For whatever delusional reason I had at the time, I believed that because of my dedication and honest investment of time spent on religious acts, I could have my champion:

> ♥A partner willing to dance for joy in the light of the Spirit, and in a life of committed love with me, forever. A partner that would glow in admiration and adoration and serve my tender heart— cherish me, be a source of strength and integrity, and a loving companion, through the good and bad times of life! ♥

I was so confused when my husband left me because I had been doing so much cleansing and work on myself. I really couldn't understand why God would give me the exact opposite of what I was praying for. I almost ended up going full circle, Spiritually speaking. Actually, I probably would have turned my back on God and given up the greatest

Fall lesson of my life altogether, if I hadn't had some real angels, in the form of Spiritually mature friendships that helped me keep my world together.

I found that during Fall, when Nature moves in, prepared or not, some change is going to take place, and if your world is full of toxins, be prepared. They gotta come up to come out!

♥Teaspoons of Love ♥

Every morning, my dear girlfriend (and ironically, my godmother) fed me little tiny teaspoons full of her personal Fall Self♥Love Potions. She had created them during a few of her own Fall life's lessons. She also knew how very powerful her potions were, and had she given me more than a teaspoon at a time, I probably would have puked it up all over the floor. So she just held my hand and said,

> *You know, God's blessings to Abraham could only be fulfilled with Sarah's cooperation. Marriage is the union of two people who become one. Not one person who becomes two! Even though your world feels like it's unraveling, continue to trust God with all your heart, my friend, and don't let your heart become hardened against your faith. You are just standing outside your comfort zone, and I guarantee you that God is standing right there with you.*

Then she would hand me the teaspoon and continue her gentle Spiritual message,

> *If you were looking for a religion that made you feel comfortable, Cynthia, I certainly would not have recommended Christianity, because Christ is always on the move, and you know what…He expects you to follow Him, wherever He leads you, my dear.*

"I came to Christ because I was looking for the truth," I replied weakly. "I just wasn't expecting to find it like this!"

I had chosen the path of faith because early on that's what I believed I was supposed to do. "Follow Him"—God that is. As my faith matured, so did my love for God and my desire to live a life that was edifying and pleasing to Him. Sure, I was going to follow Him, but that didn't make it any easier to do!

Now, in the midst of these trials, I was being reminded to keep my eye on heaven, even though I felt like I was going through hell.

I just wanted to feel good, I could have just taken a pill or had a drink. To be honest, what I really was praying for while I was in the midst of losing the very love I was trying to solidify was to just stop feeling altogether! But I kept my eye on God, and held on to my faith and the idea that somehow, tomorrow just had to be better than today.

I anchored myself heavily on my sister-in-law's early words,

You are not alone! You are not alone! You are not alone! We all have free will. You are choosing yours. Let others choose theirs.

It was hard enough trying to rely on God, but having to respect the free will of my husband during that Fall cleansing cycle was beyond my own ability at the time. It was only with the help and encouragement of the friendships I had built on a foundation of integrity, and had celebrated my life with early on, that kept me going.

♥I kept working on myself one moment, one teaspoon, one day, and one season at a time. ♥

♥ No Waste ♥

Several Falls came and went before I was really able to let go of that pain. But each season, the cleansing effect on my body, soul, and mind was made easier and easier by the new found strength this cleansing process was revealing about me.

As I continued my natural health education, I studied Nature and her seasons with intensity. I became intrigued with the rhythm and flow of Nature's cycles. I felt driven, yet inspired, to consume as much information as possible on natural healing. I had been introduced to natural health by my grandmother when I was a little girl. I learned with certainty that Mother Nature never wastes an opportunity (nor does God) and as I began to apply these theories to the facts of my life, I began to see my situation in a completely different light.

Through the eyes of Nature, I saw my life being cleansed during my pain. And here is a really fresh ♥ moment—by respecting the free will of the man I adored, and holding on to my faith while losing him, I ended up getting exactly what I had been praying for; I just didn't get it the way I had been praying for it!

> ♥ Nature was in the process of balancing and harmonizing my life and had picked the middle of Fall to do it. ♥

I found myself face to face with my past, making right with my future, and I was being presented with opportunities to help me see beyond the appearance of lack of love in my life *to a deeper, never-ending supply of eternal, authentic love.* Yes, the very thing I had been praying for. I can't say I can prove it, but I believe this as fact today: the final October of my marriage was when I experienced the greatest lesson in faith through a cleansing cycle of love.

♥ Grace

By accepting that much needed lesson in Grace, I've been able to experience some of the purest joys in the smallest moments of my life since. Accepting the free will of others with Grace is Self♥Love Potion ingredient number four, and now is a good time to do that exercise.

 ## Self♥Love Potion Ingredients

#1 ♥ *Spirituality. Your personal connection to a higher power.*
#2 ♥ *Knowing your Truths and accepting responsibility.*
#3 ♥ *Letting go of envy.*
#4 ♥ *Accepting the free will of others with Grace.*

♥ Self♥Loving Hurdles

Trying to have a relationship with a husband who didn't want to be a husband to me anymore was a painful experience for sure, and the lessons it took to get it all straightened out lead me to the most difficult crossroad of my life.

Fortunately, I was already on the path of faith, which leads to authentic Self♥Love, the kind of Self♥Loving that that has a calm potency to it. It had lain silent within me for more than three decades. Now I am able to experience more unconditional and authentic love than I could have ever worked out in a fantasy relationship that lacked reciprocal love from a man who didn't want to be there.

♥ Self♥Loving didn't happen right away ♥

I still had a few hurdles to jump along that lesson's pathway. But the fact is, I've since learned that I am truly worthy of love and was worthy of love all along.

> ♥ …not because of what I could do, or give, or provide, but simply because of who I am. ♥

That's the kind of thing faith does for our sense of self, which is really Self♥Love. We are all worthy of that kind of love. We just get sidetracked, sometimes, trying to prove it to ourselves.

October 7th will forever remain a pivotal day in the process of my finding the right recipe for my ultimate Self♥Love Potion. Call me delusional, but I now refer to those struggling years of divorce as awakening treasures! And though I rarely choose to revisit those moments of genuine pain created by the deepest Fall cleansing of my life, I still embrace the lessons each moment brought with it.

Let me take a moment to clarify something, before we go on.

> ♥ I'm not saying that God or Nature *creates* divorce! ♥

No! People do! But part of honoring God and yourself is respecting the freewill of those around you. I read somewhere, ♥ *To remove the choice is to remove the love.* ♥ So, to really love someone, sometimes you have to let go of them.

God gives us choices, but it's up to us to choose; and, I think, if you didn't invite God in on the deal in the first place, there are going to be some major changes when you finally do. Any kind of change will create new choices. In a relationship, you grow and learn together, or (as in my case) grow apart.

When my husband chose to leave me, he handed me back my heart. As painful as that experience was, I still had to choose to give my heart back to God and believe that true love was possible and existed for me—just not the way I was praying for it, perhaps.

My recommendation is that you build your relationships with God's awesome power "already" in place. That way, when the Fall season cleansing cycle comes up, year after year, you're prepared to withstand the elements, and work with them, instead of against them.

♥ Another View

That beautiful word picture, entitled *His vision of her,* that began this chapter, was written for me by a dear writer friend of mine. I have always enjoyed seeing my life in his images. His view of me is so very different than my own, which is why I think I like them so much. It's tough to think of myself as the beautiful, carefree creature he creates in his stories. I think, as a rule, others usually do see us differently than we see ourselves. But, one thing "Wordman" and I do agree on is the essential nature of my love for hearth and home. If you want to know where I truly celebrate my life, the answer you'll get will be "my home."

Home, to me, means a family of individuals singing different notes, but with the same music sheet. Even if you are single, you still have a home and family. It's those people with whom you share your life. It could be as removed as a co-worker, or as close as an intimate friendship, blood-relative, child, or love interest.

Celebrating life within your family is like putting syrup on your pancakes—it just tastes better. If you add a little flavor of "an attitude of determination and acceptance," you've got yourself a great recipe for love-tolerance syrup.

Now, I realize no marriage is perfect—nor is any person, child, spouse, or friend—but creating loving tolerance where you celebrate your life will aid you in consistently transforming a difficult situation into something beautiful.

The question is,

> ♥ Where do you find the determination to make love work? ♥

Or where would you find the desire to accept with faith, or simply to love unconditionally, if you weren't lucky enough to have had that recipe passed down to you during your childhood?

♥ Sharing Our Own Love

Certainly, learning how the other person views you and sharing your view of them is important, but I believe it's the sharing of our own Self♥Love that holds it all together. A little low on Self♥Love? So was I. The reason was because I thought I DID have an attitude of determination and acceptance. But, guess what I forgot to take into consideration: the fact that each of us has freewill.

> ♥ It is was an attitude of control when I didn't consider my partner's freewill. ♥

That little attitude of determination can turn right around and become and attitude of control! No matter how clear "MY" view was on how my life should go, the picture of the way life should go for the person sitting across from me wasn't always in line with the picture they had for themselves.

Free will is a person's right to choose the picture they want to see, and to color it with the crayons they want to use.

♥We can hand out the colors, but we can't make another person draw our picture♥

Accepting responsibility for my own actions, and respecting the free will of those around me was a very important Self♥Love Potion ingredient, one that required me to learn how to speak with honesty in my heart, and listen for the honesty spoken from the hearts of those I love. I guess Nature figured Fall was as good a time as any to start the process. I had to start with figuring out my own needs before I went around demanding they be met by anyone else. I also had to learn the subtle difference between demanding and determined.

♥Gentle

Even Nature gives warning signs that Fall is moving in. She is gentle in turning the green leaves to golden hues of yellow and red. She tints the air with a crisp whisper of her impending truths before the cool season blows in.

Once I had confidence in my convictions, I had to be responsible for the actions that followed, and respectful of the free will of those around me, as I shifted.

♥Keeping my eye on heaven and trusting in my faith allowed me to be less wishy-washy about my own boundaries, thus allowing me to give up the need to control others.♥

By letting my yeses be yes, and my nos be no, I wasn't just stirring up a bunch of old ashes from a dead Fall fire, and I wasn't as tempted to act like kerosene on a burning one, either. (The autumn winds make such a mess out of indecision.)

Gently shifting with Nature's seasons, accepting responsibility, respecting free will, drawing boundaries, and being clear, made it easier for me to listen and learn. Yeah, we have to listen, too! Darn it, huh? Listening is Self♥Love Potion ingredient number five. Let's do that exercise now.

 Self♥Love Potion Ingredients

#1 ♥*Spirituality. Your personal connection to a higher power.*
#2 ♥*Knowing your Truths and accepting responsibility.*
#3 ♥*Letting go of envy.*
#4 ♥*Accepting the free will of others with Grace.*
#5 ♥*Listening.*

♥ Listen for What's Being Said, Not Just What You Want to Hear

It became clear that life was not just all about me. I know, I know, but at least I tried to help the other person *THINK* it's not just all about me, anyway…(Wink.) I learned to listen with my whole mind, body, and Spirit for feedback; not just what I wanted to hear, but what was really being said. For every word of criticism I gave (and there were lots), I tried to offer several more in encouragement.

Since my divorce, I've had to end a few toxic relationships myself, and when I did, I tried to provide all the reasons why that person should have great success with someone else in their future.

It wasn't always easy to understand the other person's perspective, and trying to be patient in my communications was difficult, at best, but the point is, I tried. Sometimes people were just not prepared for me to blow in my cool temperature. But, remembering how I felt when it happened to me helped me offer more patience to others. At least I tried to give them time to grab a sweater.

I learned that Fall was not the time to be making big impressions or fancy statements. Speaking clearly and simply is what usually worked best. I would start small using simple easy, and clear words, and then I'd (try) to sit back and listen. Taking that time, plus a few moments to be honest with myself, helped me to honestly listen to others, too.

> ♥ I know this much: you can't move on to another relationship until you go through the one you're in. ♥

My Grammy used to say, "You're not done until you're done."

My prayer is that you're in committed relationships before God, and that your relationships can withstand a little Fall cleansing. I wish no one would ever see the end of their relationships (perhaps one day in heaven?), but my point is, if you're dating, if you have a boyfriend or girlfriend and you do want out, wait until you're really done. If you get out too soon, before you're really done, it's going to feel like you're dragging rotting parts of your current relationship into the new one with you. And you know what they say:

> ♥ It only takes one bad apple to spoil a whole bunch of good ones. ♥

Nature gives the Fall season three full months to do cleansing and harvesting, so take her advice, don't rush it. You might ask God to define that timetable for you. Don't give up, or give in, too soon. Even though love needs to flow in both directions for it to flourish,

> ♥ *True* love endures *all* things, even a good Fall cleansing! ♥

Chapter Four

Chapter Four

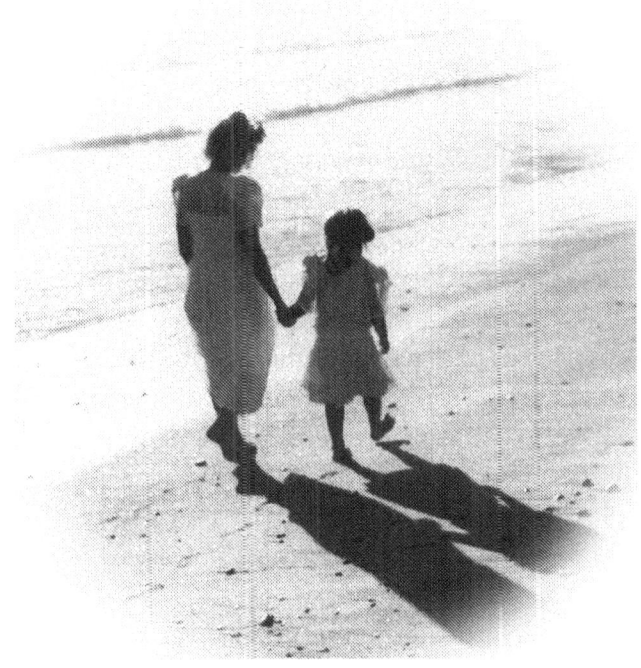

♥*A Loving Voice~*

I will always give you my best, and not just in a way to try to impress you with myself, but I want to impress 'in' you a Love that is real and is given freely.

~Authentic Acceptance

Get your priorities in order, my expression revealed, as I placed the Starbuck's on the table between us.

I stopped moving only long enough to see if I'd gotten the message across gracefully. I realized she was paying close attention when I spoke, even if she pretended to act disinterested. I knew she was eager for my insights, so I was careful not to allow her to assume too much by my silence.

There are those who have told her they considered my intuitions to be way beyond the norm, but she was the type that had to prove things to herself, and not take advice too easily.

So many times she wanted to walk away from our conversations, but our Spirit was linked in such a way, she always remained.

"What slays me about you is your audacity," she said as she took her stand in front of the table, her feet shoulder's-width apart.

She is a strong-willed, yet fragile young lady, with muscular arms and calves, certainly equipped to run or fight. The funny thing is, if she only knew that the pleasure I take away from these moments with her leaves me in such agreement with Nature's divine plan, she would never have need to quarrel for her position, anyway.

As I've watched her grow, over the years, I've come to realize she never did have the intention of fighting. She just liked being prepared. That is just her way.

"How is it you think you know me so well?" she asked, finally taking a seat beside me.

The truth be known, my words are spoken from such an unconditional love and concern for my subject, that I am hardly able to contain the expressions inside.

But, instead, I put on my intellectual mask and reply, "Well darlin', I look at what you do, not at what you say, and then I just pray for the words to come out right. Now, are you going to sit down here and tell me what's going on?"

Within the hour, she is predictably returned to composure, as she let my words and images play upon her senses.

For me, these moments with her return me to my true self. For her, it is uniquely different, but nonetheless, just as important.

As she rose to gather her things from the table, she flashed me that impish smile. No cash payment was necessary; it was all there in the twinkling of her eyes.

Half-way out the door, she stopped. Turning on one heel, she expressed the full potential of those muscular calves, as they instantly moved her across the floor.

She slid her fight-ready arms around my neck and whispered in my ear,

"Thank you, Mommy. I love you."

~C

♥The Spring in Nature's Steps ♥

♥Spring is one of my favorite times of year, and I can't think of a better example of Spring's Spirit than the sheer determination of a teenager's will. The creative energy of a teenager and the essence of Spring just seem to go hand in hand.

Spring seems to be a time to absorb the nutrients from life, and to begin planning and building dreams. I've always found that the ideas I've planted in the fertile soil of Spring generally blossom into a forceful explosion of energy during the hot months of Summer, just ahead.

Whenever I am talking with God, and my daughter is listening to my prayers, it gives me another way in which to love and communicate love to her.

> ♥I find my Springtime prayers generally turning to planning and discernment. ♥

Journaling after prayer really helps me understand what's going on inside of me. Sometimes I will just open up my mouth after praying and journaling, and the right words just flow right out!

Journaling helps me get clarity from my moments alone with myself, and once I have clarity I can more effectively share those insights with my daughter or any one else who cares to listen.

After journaling I find that I am able to have courage when my little one has fear; when she has doubt, I have confidence; when she feels weak, I am there to be her strength.

> ♥ And when her dreams seem like they are out of reach, the right words seem to be there to lift her up.

I find journaling to be such an important part of my self communication that I have made it the sixth ingredient in my Self♥Love Potion. Teaching our brains to work for us through journaling.

 # Self♥Love Potion Ingredients

#1 ♥*Spirituality. Your personal connection to a higher power.*
#2 ♥*Knowing your Truths and accepting responsibility.*
#3 ♥*Letting go of envy.*
#4 ♥*Accepting the free will of others with Grace.*
#5 ♥*Listening.*
#6 ♥*Journaling.*

~

♥A Journalized Moment♥

I was going through an old journal and realized that Springtime with my daughter is unlike any other time of the year. This is the time of year I refer to as her "teenage Spirit of adventure." Although every moment with my teenager counts to me, somehow I see her grow even more radiant and active than normal during Spring.

Spring is a time of building and planning. In Nature, we see the little seedlings sucking up the nutrients from the soil and the flowers dancing in the brilliant sunlight. Spring is on the opposite end of Fall. Spring is growth, Fall is harvest. Spring is nourishing, Fall is cleansing.

I delight in being a parent during Spring, as my daughter shares her plans, projects, strategies, convictions, and opinions of how she is going to go about making her future visions a reality. She has got to be the most precious gift of Nature I will ever personally experience. The love I have for her is way beyond any physical limitation I could ever imagine.

Of course, I am sure every mother feels like this about her own child; you can witness that same kind of love expressed between Mother Nature and her willful garden of small, flowering children during Spring, as well.

You know the kind of love I'm talking about. It flows authentically and endlessly. If you don't have a child of your own, picture the way a little one responds to the loving call of someone they recognize,

"Come here, honey."

Watch them run, their little faces turning bright with smile, arms open full-width's length, those little legs and diapered butts running straight toward the arms of the one who calls their name. It's beautiful to both watch and experience.

> ♥ Little children know no other way than to love and live from the purest parts of who they are. ♥

They freely express and experience life from its authentic and most beautiful state. It is as fresh and pleasing to behold as the Spring's morning sunrise.

But, just as the sun rises, so must it set. With each passing year, a child's Spring energy shifts and changes, until the pure and innocent, the authentic acceptance, has given way to the "teenage Spirit of adventure"—you know, that teenage discovery zone.

Some parents find it more and more difficult to communicate authentically with the purest parts of their kids during this cycle. One of the reasons, I believe, is because today's teenagers are being encouraged to hide their authentic, Spring attitudes from the world. They are taught to fear their honest passions for life and hide them behind layers and layers of masks.

~Masks of Teenage Confusion~

Contrary to the perfectionist disposition of the mother that I am, I try to encourage my daughter's Spring Spirit-of-adventure attitude. It's like the free will of Springtime ragweed. It pops up everywhere, beautiful, but is a weed nonetheless.

I confess, some of my daughter's Spring ideas have caused me a great many sleepless nights, but I think my support really empowers her self-esteem and self-worth. Conversely, I see so many of her teenage friends feeling just the opposite during these changes in their lives. Instead of growing strong through parental encouragement, I see these kids grow confused and afraid, simply because these "Spring" ideas may be in conflict with what their friends or parents perceive or expect them to be. So these kids learn to put on masks, to hide from fear of rejection.

> ♥ In doing so, they cover up the most precious parts of who they really are. They may even forget those precious parts altogether! ♥

I try my best to communicate honestly and sincerely with my daughter, and to maintain an open line of two-way communication. My hope is to avoid the problems that come along with the wearing of masks, because we all wear them. Consciously, or unconsciously, it's unavoidable.

As my daughter searches out the different faces she wants to show the world, I've tried to maintain an environment where she can always feel confident to return to the core of who she is when speaking with me.

Being available to her for these moments of authentic conversation allows her the freedom to dream big, while feeling safe enough to share her teenage Spirit and experiences, honestly, with me.

Now, some of these conversations can leave me feeling like I need an emotional Heimlich maneuver, for sure, but they also allow me to participate in the truth of who she is. Spring is like that for the world.

♥ Spring Dreams ♥

I love observing my daughter as she dreams and creates. She discovers her full potential during Springtime, and it's a refreshing perspective of life I experience when I watch her soar above the world's censored viewpoint like that.

When she inappropriately implements one of her fabulous Spring ideas, I am careful to remind her that, although my love for her is not contingent upon her pleasing me, for every choice she makes, there are going to be consequences.

> ♥Oh, so many times, when I was growing up, I thought if I did it wrong, my parents would stop loving me. ♥

That was a life lesson in how to become a people-pleaser and one lesson I didn't need to pass on to my daughter.

Fortunately, my daughter understands the concept of Grace, as God offers it to us, and I offer it to her. She knows that she could never do anything so bad that it would destroy my natural-born love for her. I think this is one of the reasons she feels safe to respectfully explore the boundaries of her teenage Spirit of adventure.

♥Mom vs. Friend♥

It's more attractive, at times, to be my daughter's friend than her parent, and sometimes it's probably easier, too; but I'm quick to remind myself that she already has plenty of friends. What she has only one of is a mother, and that's what she needs me to be.

I maintain the right to accept or reject her actions, while offering her enough encouragement and opportunity to make mistakes, with the knowledge that I will always be there for her when the going gets tough, though not always with a smile.

I think it's that kind of knowing that helps her to become more accountable with her decision-making, and allows her the security to live, authentically and responsibly, at the same time.

The wearing of masks is a tricky thing for a teenager. It's tricky for us all. As a matter of fact, that is Self♥Love Potion ingredient number seven: Identifying the many masks we wear.

 # Self♥Love Potion Ingredients

#1 ♥*Spirituality. Your personal connection to a higher power.*
#2 ♥*Knowing your Truths and accepting responsibility.*
#3 ♥*Letting go of envy.*
#4 ♥*Accepting the free will of others with Grace.*
#5 ♥*Listening.*
#6 ♥*Journaling.*
#7 ♥*Identifying Masks, revealing your true nature.*

♥True Nature♥

Some of us have been wearing masks for so long that we have lost touch with the authentic Spirit underneath. The question is, are you willing to show your true nature? You have to be in order to have a meaningful relationship with someone else.

Relationships start from the center of who we are; if we have hidden that center under layers and layers of masks, we may find it difficult to access and express clearly.

Remember when I suggested:

> ♥ If we are unclear as to our own needs, we are going to have a much more difficult time communicating them to another person. ♥

We can end up feeling as if we are faking it in a relationship, which can lead to hurt feelings and eventually, anger, simply because we were unable to communicate an expectation clearly. It can even lead to getting or giving forged affection.

♥ Fair Share of Advice ♥

Being an authentic single parent, with issues of my own to deal with, can be…well…quite treacherous at times. I sought out my fair share of professional advice the year my husband left me. It was a tenuous time for living authentically with a teenager, trying to decide when to let my daughter really see my authentic pain and weakness, and when to wear my parent's mask of strength, for love's sake.

Somehow, in Nature's great wisdom, the year she and I shared that spaghetti dinner in the middle of the floor in our empty living room apartment, turned out to be the fertilizer for some of the deepest, richest moments and conversations of our mother-daughter teenage experience so far.

I was so afraid the term "dysfunctional family" would be stamped across her forehead, forever! Fortunately, my counselor kept me from worrying myself to death about things I had no control over, and she gave me some great wisdom I'll share with you now.

She said that the amount of time, money, and energy I put into healing myself then was going to pay off tenfold in the life of my daughter, later on.

She was so right. I can already see benefits of that labor of Self ♥ Love.

♥ Benefits to a Labor of Love

"Do you still love him, Mom?" my daughter asked, seeing me wipe the tear that was forming in the corner of my eye.

"Ah, honey, these old memories have to come up to come out. This is just the way my body is making room inside for some great, new experience," I say as I'm sifting through some old pictures.

Noticing her silence, I continue, "To answer your question—No, I'm no longer in love with the man; but I am still in love with the fantasy of who I thought he could be in my life, and that's what hurts so much, honey. I will probably always miss that part of our relationship, sweetie. But these little Spring tears are making some extra room in my heart for God's perfect love. See, people may let you down from time to time, because they are not perfect. But God's love is, and always will be there for us, because it is perfect," I add, softening my answer by respectfully placing a picture of her and her daddy amongst those of her friends, on her bedroom picture shelf.

"We have quite an exciting life ahead of us Peaches, wouldn't you agree?" I say, with a reassuring smile and a kiss on the cheek.

With a mirthful smile in return, she kisses me back and hands me a handful of left-over candy corns.

Satisfied for the moment, she turns on a dime and skips out of the room. Absolutely priceless!

♥ Gentle but Deliberate ♥

Nature has a gentle but deliberate Spirit and will never give you more than you can handle. It may not always feel so, but it's true. I've become quite friendly with that little fact of Nature.

> ♥ The body will only bring up and eliminate what it can tolerate at the time. ♥

So, each year, each season, the past makes way for the future, and it gets easier and easier to let go. Spring is a great time to lay out those future plans. If you have a teenager, you'll need several Springs to plan for what comes next. I can't even recall the number of hours I've spent preparing my speech for the day I would need to lay it on the boy who would even think about spending any quality time with my little (now seventeen-year-old) angel.

Oh, it was quite exciting creating the plan for exactly how I would get my point across, convincingly. Mind you, I am only five feet tall and weigh little more than 105 lbs. The boys in my daughter's ninth grade class out-sized me almost by half. So, I figured I was going to have to prepare myself for the day one of them would come a callin.'

♥ The Invitation ♥

I imagined inviting the young man into the house and strategically standing him within pointing distance of a picture I had hung on the wall—the one of a tiny pink dress enclosed within the grasp of a 6'4", 264lb ex-bodybuilding father's ominous arms.

I would then proceed to explain how precious my little girl is to me, and the fact that, although her daddy wouldn't be going on the date with them, that didn't mean that her Father wasn't.

Then, I'd step back, just enough to let the bewildered-looking young man catch a glimpse of the aforementioned picture, hanging right next to that of a cross.

I would continue on to explain that I was talking about her Father in heaven, and inquire, without really waiting for a reply, "You do know God, don't you?"

At this point I would assume the young man would be overwhelmed with conflicting emotions on how to answer me, and my implied message would hit the bulls-eye.

"See him?" I'd say, pointing to her dad's picture. "Can you imagine how dangerous it would be to make him angry? Well multiply that by about 100,000 times and you'll get an idea of how unwise it might be for you to put one of our HEAVENLY Father's favorite daughter's best interests or safety at risk this evening."

This guilt technique is a little something I learned from my ritualistic, Spiritual experiences…(wink).

Anyway, then I would wait for the young man's response (and presumably the color to return to his face). Then I'd add, "I believe God is even more protective of His children than I could ever hope to be, so I am assuming I am making myself clear?"

After that, I'd re-ask him where it was he said they were going for the evening while offering him a fresh baked cookie from my oven. With a smile, of course.

Oh man, I had it all planned out in my head, exactly how it was going to go down. It was absolutely perfect until I tried it out for the first time. This guy showed up as authentically prepared with an answer as I was with my plan. Smart kids they're making these days!

No matter though, I'm sure that by offering my daughter the opportunity to live with the knowledge of God's authentic love for her, it's given her an incredible sense of security and independence.

Even if she won't admit it to my face. I know in my heart of hearts that if something ever happened to me, she is strong willed and self-actualized enough to really make it in this world and live a life of balance and peace.

She truly understands the important roles faith and God play in her life. That understanding gives her courage to stand up for what she believes in, as well as to share her wisdom with others. Her friends turn to her for answers when they can't find answers themselves.

> ♥ Her guidance is always smooth—not always gentle, but very matter of factly, and unarguably clear. ♥

She is a mentor of sorts to friends years older than her. When I ask her about it, she blows it off as simply a duty of friendship. But I watch her put herself in their place as she offers herself up genuinely. I'd like to take credit for the gift she writes off to friendship, but I know this wisdom does not come from me. It's a gift from God himself to one of his darling daughters. As I watch hardened hearts open to her as trustingly as a blooming flower unfolds to Spring's inspired plan, I am once again reminded what it is like

> ♥ To serve life and love authentically, without hesitation. ♥

Spring has that way about it, too. It's a time to serve the desires of my heart without hesitation.

An Empowering Moment

♥ Several seasons after my divorce, while I was still swimming around in a stagnant pool of my own self pity, Spring ventured in close and blew her version of a building message into my broken heart. It turned out to be quite an empowering moment of deep self-worth when I finally understood the plan and eventually accomplished the goal.

I stood there looking out over the greatness of the ocean from my second-story balcony. Spring began to sing her inspiring message as her breath carried my hair away from my face.

Why are you waiting for a Mr. Right to give you a ring in order to remove the painful ghosts of your past? Build one for yourself from the pleasant memories of your history and let it serve as a beacon of your own Self ♥ Love. Hold fast to your faith that God has a plan for your life and your painful ghosts will fade like the ocean's mist gives way to an amber sunset or rising sun.

Standing there a moment longer I caught a whiff of Spring's wild-flowers. I assessed how long had it been since I had blessed myself with a planned gift of Self♥Love and nurturing. Ahhh, Self♥Love portion ingredient number eight! Blessing yourself with a symbol of Self♥Love. Once you realize you're worthy to receive your own gifts of love, it makes the receiving of those gifts momentous occasions to cherish.

 **Self♥Love Potion Ingredients**

#1 ♥*Spirituality. Your personal connection to a higher power.*
#2 ♥*Knowing your Truths and accepting responsibility.*
#3 ♥*Letting go of envy*
#4 ♥*Accepting the free will of others with Grace.*
#5 ♥*Listening.*
#6 ♥*Journaling.*
#7♥*Identifying Masks, revealing your true nature.*
#8 ♥*Symbols of Self♥Love.*

~

♥A Meaningful Symbol♥

It had been too long since I had taken the time to do a little something for me. That's when I set my mind to the preparation of a wearable symbol of Self♥Love that would express value for my life's choices—the good and the bad ones! Something that would represent the fact that I was ready to let go of my past pains and reclaim the positive from them. I wanted to make amends for the harm I had done to myself esteem and create an inspiring foundation for my future.

So what I did first was go to my jewelry box full of sentimental love offerings, where I had kept locked away all of those haunting symbols of my past. Since I had been too emotionally fragile to wear any of these gifts, for fear of resurrecting the pain I had associated with them, I kept them tucked away out of sight.

There they were, sitting untouched, locked up, a prisoner to my own meaning, magnifying the ghostly feelings of my past like an old graveyard full of head plates. Was I about to resurrect all the pain I had buried inside this box?

This was going to take some careful planning, I thought to myself.

Then I began the vigilant process of choosing stones that captured the truth of the offering without resurrecting the ghost of the giver.

First I chose a large Emerald stone and remembered the day my husband had given it to me. He knew how much I loved emeralds, and he wanted to please me one holiday. Mind you, we had just finished funding our first chiropractic office and first new home together. It was a financially tenuous time for us both; nonetheless, he bartered and finagled and next thing I new, I was opening the box to one of the most beautiful emeralds I could have ever dreamed of. It was one of the first "major" gifts of jewelry I ever received from him, besides my engagement ring, and it held significant emotional value to me, as it was a true offering of love and genuine symbol of motherhood.

A perfect place to start! I thought.

> ♥ Rather than focusing on the loss of the man who gave it to me, I decided to use this symbol as a positive reminder of who I was as a dedicated & loving mother. ♥

With the help of the cool Spring breeze reminding me to "prune the memories," the next question was to figure out what to surround this bright green symbol of parenthood with.

Hmmmm—I could choose the cracked and damaged pearl…or the diamond that my mom gave me from my daddy's ring, or the garnet from the ring my daughter won in a poetry contest in eight grade….No, that one was still wearable as is! Let's see, there was the actual wedding ring of my innocence. No, that won't do. I'm not quite so innocent any-more. How about the gold band, twisted into the name "Simba."

So on and on it went, until finally my mind had become so exhausted and I just laid there on my bedroom floor listening to the sound of Springs songbirds outside my window. Animated love songs rode the ocean airwaves in though my open door.

I sat up to get a closer look at the little sound vessels and stretched my leg up over my jewelry box to have a look out the window. Missing my stretch, I knocked over the entire jewelry box.

Chains and trinkets scattered everywhere as the box tumbled to its side. Underneath the red velvet hinge I saw the tip of a piece of white paper. As I pulled it from beneath its resting-place, a soothing Spring breeze comforted my mind, like the familiar smell of cookies. The note read:

…this present time cannot be compared at all with the glory that is going to be revealed…Remember, you will never be deserted by God, so have the faith to look beyond the appearance of lack and see a never-ending supply of God!

Spring was once again reminding me not to treat this work of love so cerebrally.

♥ I had to let go of my artificial defense and get back to the plan. ♥

Listening to the songs of love from outside my window, each gem began singing as well. God did have a plan for my life and these gems represented some of the stop signs along the way.

♥ Just as the songbirds were building their nest, I was building the voice of my future. ♥

And my future belonged to God, of that I was sure. In that moment I settled on six white diamonds from the band of my engagement ring. I choose them to remind me of the many rewards I had received on the road I traveled as a wife, as well as the many lessons I had learned.

I wasn't giving up on the hope that dedicated love was still possible for me. Those very lessons would shine a light on the path God intended me to travel in my future and remind me what NOT to do next time.

One day my daughter will have this ring and the story that goes along with it. I wanted it to last, so I had the stones set in platinum squaring the bottom of the band, to signify a firm foundation, and lined the six diamonds evenly on either side of the emerald.

Perfect, I thought.

I thanked the songbirds for their musical distraction. And silently I said a prayer of thanksgiving to the writer of the hidden note. Once the setting had been completed, I took it to my place of worship and asked a blessing be placed upon it. This act was another symbol to me, that I was moving forward.

It was then suggested that I create my own blessing to be used in conjunction with the traditional sanctioning.

Ok, I thought, so I took out my old journal and fashioned this prayer from my thoughts and feelings past.

Lord, I ask You to help me forgive those who have hurt me, and I release those offenders to Your will. Because I need forgiveness as well, I ask You to help me make amends, in a peaceful way, to those whom I have harmed, consciously or otherwise. I offer my life and my future to You and I ask that my actions and my very life be used as a witness to Your existence, and that my pain and triumphs would become inspiration to the hearts of others. Take my anger, pain, and suffering Lord, and make them like the rainbows after a flood in this ring's reflection. I earnestly believe that You exist and that I matter to You, so I ask that You would help me to see Your pure light and purpose for my future.

Spring's plan had been revealed and implemented. Its design was to help me discover that I was worth the creating and the giving of this symbol of love to myself. I felt like a teenager all over again, living in authentic communication with myself.

> ♥The rewards for that kind of effort go far beyond a Mr. Right with a diamond of any size!♥

Chapter Five

Chapter Five

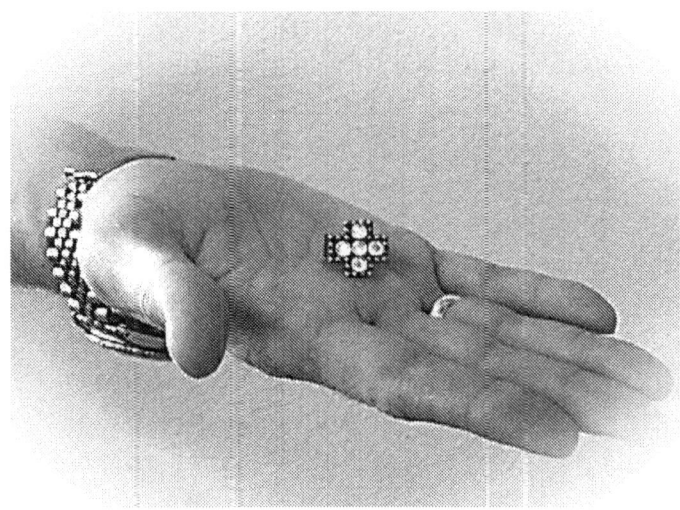

♥ A Loving Voice~

Everything God gives to me, and that which I work for, is not a tool to be used to win you, and then bed you, and keep you wanting. It is my mission to let God love you through me, and see that you are truly happy from within.

~ The Parade

Smoothly and skillfully, he put her at ease, magnifying their friendship with polite conversation and genuine laughter.

Although his cool nature confused her, she admired his intelligence and adored his sensitivity even more. He was a man accustomed to being pursued, and she, a woman used to the same.

She fell onto the bed next to him and smiled at his reaction to her, as he reached up to straighten his shirt collar and crossed his heavy-soled shoes atop the blue and white bedspread, while clearing his throat.

He was a practical man, a somber mind with understandable temperaments. He was a man that had to stay in control. Some might say he was arrogant, but she knew that was just his way.

He drew his strength (not to Fall for her) from the distraction of the passing parade, outside, not so much for her heart's sake, but for his. His was a heart that would need nudging.

She was careful to draw boundaries with him, yet gave him great latitude to maneuver, because she saw his need for time, space and healing. She also knew that her own life's lesson in heart's abandonment was to wait on God, so she was committed to developing more patience with the call of chemical romantic attraction. And, so…she remained silent to what she felt happening between them, that night.

He could feel it, too; that particularly paralyzing feeling of vulnerability and strength, like a swiftly burning candle within him.

He stopped for a moment to listen to the music from the parade, passing outside the window. The music reminded him that he had skills sufficient to please her. Still, he was struggling with that uneasy feeling of vulnerability she evoked within him.

There is something different about this girl, he thought.

She was tugging at the very heart of him. That's what he feared most about her, her desire for commitment. Or was it his? He sensed the physical passion between them.

Tonight it would be easy to challenge her boundaries. He thought, considering his options, and then cautioning himself that she may deny him, again.

She was aware that he had a great appetite for sex. She too, if committed, shared his need. She was also thoughtful of his thirst for "the beautiful women," which gave her considerable satisfaction, being one he would consider worthy of the pursuit. It also made it a frustrating proposition to refuse him. But she desired God's blessings in her relationship more than the exhilaration of the chemistry they shared.

She bit her lip and sighed, as she watched the shadows dance upon the bedroom wall from the parade passing outside her window. Her hunger was for true love, a bliss she was beginning to trust in, once again; the kind of bliss that only comes from a pledge, shared between two people, in God's name, she believed, anyway.

The world has a funny way of keeping hearts closed, she thought to herself, drawing in a deep breath.

One big continual parade of choices out there; a prettier make, a flashier trophy, a tempting alternative, she mused, as she ran the palm of her hand over the cotton flower-print pillowcase, letting out a sigh.

I hate that annoying, meddlesome parade! she thought, flashing her doe-like eyes up at him, smiling and praying that, one day, she could somehow make that distracting, incessant music stop.

Hearing her sigh, he extended his athletic arms, inviting her toward comfort, but perceptive to the fact that he could rely on her better than she could him.

Touching her face, he softly brushed the highlighted trails of hair from her cheeks. Soothing the crease from her forehead, he studied the movement of her eyes, and watched the wheels and tumblers turning and clicking in her brain. He knew that look, but he didn't dare ask the questions.

She lowered her eyes and turned her back into him, offering him her contours, as he continued to explore the lines of her neck and shoulder.

She is the eternal optimist, he smiled, as he traced the small of her back with his fingertip, secure in that tonight, if he asked, she would not deny him again. He knew he was her weakness, and she knew it, too.

Longing to let her guard down in his arms, she drew in a deep breath and felt safe enough to nestle even closer to him. Though continuing to demand diligence and truth, she allowed herself the pleasure of comfort and protection, lying there in his arms. She also offered him access to her heart.

Aware of the trust she placed within his grasp, he kissed her, softly at first. His lips gently explored her skin, sending shivers down her spine. She arched her back, feeling his breath on her neck.

Oh please, let him be your very best for me, God, she whispered into the evening air.

And there were more prayers.

Your will Lord, not mine, she uttered, silently, as his arms gently pulled her closer to him, into his chest, into his world and away from her thoughts.

He could feel her conflicted, as he cautiously turned her toward him. Her scent filled his consciousness, and he paused for a moment to watch her breathe before he kissed her, full, hard, and deep upon her lips. His heart began racing as if it were going to leap from his very chest, and he could feel himself struggling to maintain his own composure. He began reaching for control, but it was too late. Somehow, she had already opened him up. Seeing his own reflection in her eyes, he stopped to watch her breath, while taking a moment to steady his own. Now he was conflicted, in emotion and desire.

How does she do this to me? he thought, pulling himself back.

There, in her eyes, he was seeing himself in a way no woman had ever made him see himself, before. *Will this feeling still be here in the morning?* he wondered, as he reached for the window above her head, letting in the cool ocean breeze and the music from the strutting parade, outside the window. Returning his gaze to hers, he once more considered his options. The music grew louder outside the window, distracting him, confusing him, and reminding him of the dangers associated with commitment and love's promise, if he went there with her.

With her, I'd have to be a better man than I am on my own, he considered, heeding the music.

But, she also gives you the desire to want to be that kind of man for her, his Spirit countered.

She watched the expressions of his internal struggle, as he looked deep into her eyes. She smiled at his efforts to regain control.

Lord, don't let me be just another timeout from the parade for him. Love him through me, she delicately mouthed, looking up at him. She knew his heart may never belong to any woman, but she had hope. As she made her plea to God, believing she could become a force of good with him, there in her own little portion of the universe, another night of choices unfolded between them.

Then, morning came. Stretching her arms high above her Head, peace and quiet filled the room, like the light of the rising sun on the first day of Summer.

Something is different, she thought, wiping the sleep from her eyes. *The music—the shadows.*

Blinking her eyes several times, she pulled back the white linen curtains to take a closer look.

"Oh, God, we did it!" she whispered, confirming what her heart was struggling to believe. "Look! We did it; we truly and actually did it!" Not realizing how true the words, "Oh, God," actually were, she continued to rub her eyes in disbelief.

As the end result of each of their choices harmonized in the still morning air, she began to shake. When she could no longer contain her excitement, she squealed with delight, jumping up and down on the bed, looking around the room for the object of her heart's affection.

It stopped! Gone, all of them! The people the parade, the noise, it's finally gone. We finally made the right choice, and now all of those annoying, distracting women, they are all finally gone!

As her feet tangled with the bed spread, slowing her leaps of joy, she realized that not only had the parade departed, so had he.

The reality was, they had each made choices in the night that had set in motion further choices for the other.

Although he had grown by the knowing of her, it was there, at that crossroad of love's promise, that his love matured. He chose not to charm her into the shallow intimacy of the perpetual parade that he had endured all his life. He knew that life would eventually destroy her if he took her there. For the first time, he cared more about her heart than his own needs. He acknowledged that making love to her would only result in taking love from her, and he was in love with her…and now, he wanted more for her.

For her, it was the choosing of authentic love over immediate love that stopped the cycle of pain, noise, and confusion. Her faith that God would heal her abandoned heart, if she would just follow His will for her life, and not her own, had finally been realized.

"I finally got it, and now I get it!" she sang, with elfin-like merriment, as she freed her footing from the tangled spread and continued to dance about the deserted room.

Now surrounded by peace, harmony, and faith, she twirled about in fascination, dancing in delight to the tune of her own music, feeling full from within and finally available to what God had had in store for her all along;

His very BEST for her…(to be continued)

~C

♥ The Wildfires of Summer, and, Man, oh Man…Men!

♥ Impatience is the hardest of lessons to lick, and such a childish thing, don't you think? Ahhh, but then, I'm quick to remind myself of all those hot, Summer, chemistry-filled lessons I would have had to miss out on if I hadn't been such a child!

Oh, the sweet and sour flavor of Summer's chemistry is enough to make your mouth pucker at just the thought. This is the time of year for movement, experimenting, and explosions!

With that in mind, you may just want to read this chapter twice and experience this season's love lessons vicariously, and less painfully, through me! I think that's the wisest advice I could possibly share with you, considering all the times I've tried to take matters of love into my own hands, only to end up flat on my face in the hot Summer dirt.

♥ Demanding Attention ♥

Summer ushers in her lessons of love and life on her schedule, not yours. Chemistry will demand your attention, and Mother Nature simply expects it! The rhythm demonstrated by Nature during Summer, in my opinion, defies practicality.

> ♥Summer is a chemically-charged and predictably unpredictable time of year. So, be prepared! ♥

My Self♥ Love Potions are just chock-full of sizzling Summer formulae. Even when I was married, Summertime seemed to be the time of year that I would experience the true vitality of my passions. Perhaps it's because Summer brings with it the energy of fire?

The hot Summer seasons have provided for the baking of some of the most explosive cooking disasters of my heart's kitchen, but in the Summer heat, when I got it right, I got it Cheesecake Factory right!

I was just sitting here thinking about how many Summer catastrophes I've truly created.

> ♥Certainly, the most unpalatable one was letting identical men teach me the same lessons over and over again. ♥

I guess the question that matters more than that notion is, why was I letting them?

♥The Ride Continues♥

Remember that limo ride with God I was talking about earlier? Well here is where the story really began. The only reason I had agreed to take that road trip in the limo with God in the first place was to find true love.

Now, when God gave me His guarantee that if I followed Him, I would find true love, I just assumed we were talking about the same thing. So, I got right to work and created the height, weight, hair color, shoe size, financial status, etc., of exactly what I considered to be the perfect recipe of a man for me, and I just handed that list to God and said, "Okay, this is where I want to go, take me here, and I'll follow you."

God just smiled at me and said, "I don't love you because you love me, you know?" Then He paused and looked at me as if I understood what He was trying to imply with His tonality. "I love you because of who I know you to be, and I want you to see yourself as I have always seen you."

I just stood there.

"Okay," He said, realizing I had no clue what He was talking about. "When you can see yourself like I do, that's when you will authentically know true love."

I continued starring blankly back at Him with my hand on my hip, tapping my foot impatiently.

He just shook His head and said, "Okay, get in. We're going to have to go through this lesson by lesson, it appears."

"Finally," I said, letting out my breath and climbing in to the back of the limo. "How long is it going to take me to find him, and what about my clothes? I can't meet the man of my dreams wearing this old outfit," I prattled rather pompously as He drove.

Then, Whammo! "As you designed, my dear."

"Wow!" I gasped, "That was pretty fast and almost too easy," I said with cautious gratitude. "I didn't travel with You very far. What do I owe You?"

"For now, just the broken pieces of your heart, my dear," He said with a glistening smile. "I'm just gonna hang around for a while, though, if you don't mind. You know where I'll be if you need me. Just call My Name and I'll come get you. But only if you want Me to, of course," He added, with a wink.

"Broken pieces of my heart...?" my voice trailed, eyes widening at the sight in front of me.

"Go on, little one. There is an entire room full of men with everything you asked for. I'm sure one of them will do for now," He said, pointing

with a tilt of his head. "*Go. But if you call on me, remember your promise, and don't return without your broken pieces as an offering to me.*" Then poof, He was gone.

Not paying much attention to what God had just asked of me, I agreed to His terms and waved goodbye, brushing the wrinkles from my new dress. I felt like Cinderella and He was my Fairy Godfather.

I was a little confused at first, but then my eyes focused in on what God had left behind. There was no mistaking it. I saw him before I'd even gotten out of the limo. As soon as I entered the room, I could feel his energy.

Yup, that was him; it had to be him. How could it not be?

♥ There, standing just a few feet away from me,
was the man all women dream of meeting,
and all mothers fear their daughters will. ♥

Now, I'm not into one-night stands; but if I were, this would have been the night I'd have wanted to have the experience of it! Summer was already ten steps ahead of me, with her mind-controlling Chemistry, as my eyes took in the entire range of vision.

We looked right at each other. No words were exchanged, but the chemistry was so strong that my girlfriends could see the sparks flying from across the room. Finally he managed to break his own rule and moved toward me first.

Ahhh so round one goes to the female, I smiled to myself, remembering my Grammy telling me, "Always let the man pursue you, that way you'll know he's really interested in you and wants to be the man in the relationship, instead of the little boy." Oh, my Grammy cracked me up some times.

Anyway, he speaks, and as I watch his lips moving about his sparkling white teeth and the perfectly placed laugh lines highlighting his crystalline blue eyes, I hear nothing but the music, Santana to be specific, playing in the background. My girlfriends can see what's happening and try to save me from myself by warning me to "stay away from that one." But do I listen. NO! I continue to revel in the combustion happening between us.

Now mind you, on a cool Winter's day, I'm sure I'm not even this guy's type, but for some reason—chemistry, my fabulous magnetic charm, or maybe God's plan to teach me a whole new love lesson. Who knows?—I managed to draw this guy toward me and into a delightful conversation with a simple smile on my part.

This had to be the one, I confirmed, silently thanking God for his kindness.

Just as I was finishing my prayer of thanks, I got this vision of God just kicking back with His hands above his head, feet up on the steering wheel, smiling and reminding me of my promise to hand over my broken pieces if I wanted to go back. It felt like God was trying to tell me something in my gut.

Nah! I knew better, I finalized, closing the deal with myself. I ignored the multitude of red flags going up all over the place, both inside of me and around me.

"Sure, I'd love to!" I said throwing caution to the wind and accepting a drink and a go at the dance floor with Mr. Chemistry.

Almost instantly I became aware that this guy was not interested in a long-term, monogamous, potentially marriage-bound relationship, but the chemistry I was feeling was so overwhelming that I convinced myself *"he had potential."*

Oh, how many times had I done that before and would I still do it again?

This one will be different I persuaded myself to believe. *If I just work hard at I,* I continued. *He's just going to need a little time to realize I'm the one for him, too!* I rationalized; and by doing so, I positioned myself to be just like every other woman in his life.

But that part of the lesson wasn't realized 'til later. For now I was hell-bent on making the unpredictable stability of this guy's nature, a mellow, robust remedy that would patch together the broken pieces of my heart if I drank him down slowly. I was convinced that he was my missing ingredient!

> ♥ With him, I believed I could create the greatest love potion of all time! ♥

♥ Everything I asked? ♥

So there he was, everything I had asked for: smart, sexy, smelled good, looked good, loved to read, well-versed in music, loved good food, nice clothes, and this edge…Oh, he had this oh-so-confident edge to him!

Then of course, there was that picture I kept getting in my head of God trying to tell me something wasn't quite right. Perhaps it was just the fact that Mr. Chemistry acted as if he hid nothing, yet everything about his life was a mystery to me that caused the uneasy feeling in my gut.

Continuing to ignore the warning signs, I abandoned those caution signals and fell hook, line, and sinker for this guy immediately. I am sure I pushed the limits of God's patience with me, too, as I enjoyed the blazing Summer energy and stayed out 'til 2:00am, dancing the tie dance on a Thursday night!

I can still picture God sitting there, with His feet up on the dash, waiting for me to figure it out, knowing what I was headed for but unable to help me see it beforehand! How many times I've experienced that same "knowing, but letting her figure it out on her own" type of feeling with my own daughter. It makes me laugh, now. But at the time,

I was in chemical bliss and denial, and I thought this guy was everything I'd asked for.

♥ Effort ♥

Mr. Chemistry showed great effort and interest in the beginning. We met for coffee, Harley rides and a cruise up the coast in his Jaguar. Within the month, after spending four days at the river, he flew me up to meet his parents in Denver and invited me to do something wild: ride back to California on the back of his Harley!

Why not, I thought.

Just because I was still recovering from a major kidney and hip injury that I had sustained while horse back riding in Canada only six months earlier, and every doctor I talked to advised me not to do it, didn't mean I should give up the chance to experience a cross-country trip with the most thrilling man I had ever met. So what if my hip and kidney were gonna get bounced all over the place? If he didn't care, why should I?

> ♥*Live a little!* my chemistry shouted. ♥

Giving it little more consideration than arranging for my daughter to be cared for while I was gone (just in case), off we went, stopping in Vail, Utah, Brain's Head, and Vegas.

My chemistry blazed the trail ahead of me so intensely that my heart never took the time to separate the reality from the delusion of what was really taking place between us, nor did I take much time for prayerful discernment to figure it out, either.

> ♥ All I knew was this guy made me feel so alive, he could have persuaded me to go anywhere and do just about anything. ♥

I was so caught up in the excitement of our Summer chemistry, I hardly noticed how inconsistent his behavior was, or how capricious he was about actually spending quality time with me, before and after that trip ended. He just had this way of making my heart sing so loud whenever he was around that I didn't care.

I had ended all other potential relationships as soon as I met him. I really believed with every part of me that this was going to be the man of my dreams.

Silently thanking my husband for leaving me, I continued to ignore the red flags that were now torn into shreds from whipping around in the wind for so long.

I continued to make up excuse whenever Mr. Chemistry apologized for his absent behavior. Then I'd resort to using my self-indulgent ego to bargain.

You give first, and I'll give back, and we'd begin to fight each other for the right to be cherished.

♥ Burn & Destroy ♥

If you have any Summer history of your own behind you, you can see right where this is leading. Sizzle is great, but you know as well as I do, to continually burn means to continually destroy.

In order for him to preserve his chemical fire and feed his insatiable thirst for excitement, he constantly needed to be exposed to kindling. And it wasn't always mine!

I tried to manufacture explosive potions to keep the embers glowing, but seasons being what they are, they change with or without our permission, and I could tell that Winter was approaching fast.

Needless to say, it fell apart about as fast as it got started. As swiftly as he pursued me in the beginning, he retreated in the end. But it was too late for me by then; my heart was already revisiting abandonment's pain.

> ♥Although I thought I knew what love was, and I plainly understood the role I wanted to play as a loving, Christian woman, I was clearly struggling. ♥

Surely I must be doing something wrong (and I was), *or maybe my man-picker is just permanently broken,* I thought to myself, trying not to feel the depth of my heart's injuries. *Oh God, where did I go wrong?* I doubted, as a tear began to stream down my cheek (which is Self♥Love Potion ingredient number nine, by the way—asking for help!

 # Self♥Love Potion Ingredients

#1 ♥Spirituality. Your personal connection to a higher power.
#2 ♥Knowing your Truths and accepting responsibility.
#3 ♥Letting go of envy.
#4 ♥Accepting the free will of others with Grace.
#5 ♥Listening.
#6 ♥Journaling.
#7 ♥Identifying Masks, revealing your true nature.
#8 ♥Symbols of Self♥Love.
#9 ♥Asking for Help!

"You called, my child?" I heard a voice say.

Looking around expecting to see God actually standing right there, I heard the voice continue…

"You have a very limited perception of what it really feels like to 'be loved,' my dear," He said, invisibly. "To allow a man to love you more than he loves himself is an art, and you, my dear, have no idea what I mean by that statement yet. But that lesson is being offered to you now. The reason you continue to choose men that are unwilling to offer you the kind of love I offer the world is because you do not yet trust my love for you.

God's voice continued, gliding in on the midnight breeze as the current of air blew against my welling tears. Looking over my shoulder to see if He was standing next to me, I heard Him continue,

"A man must have a healthy concept of who I am in order to understand how to offer you this kind of love, and you must fill yourself with My love for you—Self♥Love—on a deeper level, so you can share this love between you from a healthy place within, and not the desperate need from without. Let Me ask you a question; do you believe you are worthy of the kind of love I am speaking of?"

"Ye-sss…I…I think so," I replied, softly wiping my water-soaked cheeks with the corner of my dress and continuing to look for the origin of the voice.

"I don't think you do, My dear, and that's why I am here for you. I think you will find that there are some profoundly important things missing from that "perfect man" shopping list you handed Me earlier. You are looking for the kind of love you seek in the wrong place from the wrong men. Why don't you try to follow MY will for your life, and look for the kind of love you seek from others willing to follow MY will for their lives as well," the voice put into plain words for me.

Looking out into the night air, I replied, "Look, I want to follow YOUR will for my life, but I'm struggling. I'm not sure I completely trust Your navigational skills anymore than I trust my own. I just think You've given me a permanently broken heart," I sniffled, as my eyes continued to well.

"I can understand how it may seem more painful, at times, to follow My will for your life rather than your own. I can only present you with the choices; you have to do the choosing, child. I have, however, placed a gift of healing others within you, in exchange for your pain," He said, His words coming to me on a warm wind that surrounded my shivering shoulders.

"Let's start over, shall we? Dare you believe in My promises to you? Tell Me your heart's greatest desire," he asked in such a manner that I believed He already knew with certainty my answer.

After pausing a short moment to recognize the magnitude of my self-inflicted wounds, and fearing my answer would be inept, I answered Him. "I want to feel and share real love," I said as my trembling calmed in the warm Summer breeze. "…but I don't understand why I keep making the same mistakes over and over again? If I am to follow this gift of healing others that You have given me, then don't You think You should make it easier to follow Your will over my own? Shouldn't I be happier right now? Shouldn't my life be perfect?" I said, turning my face into the circling wind. "Why don't You just tell me what to look for and what to stay away from? And how come You didn't just give me a room full of better choices to choose from in the first place! How come You left me all alone to figure all this out on my own?" I added, mumbling under my breath.

"My child, I will never leave you, even though you may feel that I have. I did give you a room full, a world full of wonderful choices, but you must do the choosing, my dear. You can't make good choices unless you understand the options, so don't be too hard on yourself. Why don't you spend a little more time reading the human user's manual I have provided for you? I think you call it the Bible? Anyway, continue to follow Me, and not only will I bring you the desires of your heart, but you will truly know love, and eventually understand why you hurt from some of the choices you've already made. Each day is a new day, and I can take anything from your past and use it for good. I will show you how to see Me in everything you do, and, when you can, I will reveal my plan for you to use the past pains in your life to heal others. Trust me!" His irresistible voice encouraged.

As I sat there crying, lips quivering, I implored God to just get me out of the mess I had made of my heart once again. Sobbing, I took a few more moments to focus on the harsh reality that, although God didn't really leave me there alone, He wasn't literally going to come back and get me out of there, either. I got into this mess by my own choices, so I was going to have to deal with the residual effects. At least I got that much out of His message.

I remembered my grandma telling me as a child, "You can't go forward to the next lesson until you go 'through' the last one, but no matter how it turns out, God can always use the broken pieces of your heart, and by His love, He can always make you whole again."

Ever grateful for my grandmother's early counsel, I began to understand what God was asking of me. I began to offer thanks for everything in my life, even the pain of my broken heart in that moment. I was actually excited about getting the lesson all worked out in my head, and I started to recall some of the important guidelines I had discounted from the user's manual God had referred to earlier. I made a promise to myself to go back and really study that book.

♥ Lust, Love & Chemistry ♥

Suddenly, a paperback fell right out of the midnight sky called *The Alchemy of Love and Lust*, by Theresa L Crenshaw, M.D. The attached note read,

Not in place of, but in addition to your commitment to study My Word, enjoy,

God

I began scanning a few of the pages. Next thing I knew, I had read the entire book.

Ahhhh, I think I get it!

Part of the problem with my immediate situation was that by my lack of discernment (not following the rules) I had placed myself in a situation that may have caused my own chemistry to turn against me.

My romantic heart was being held hostage by my own psychological misconceptions, as well as my own chemistry, which was forcing me, at the threat of great physical pain, to hang on for Mr. Chemistry just a little while longer every time he said he was going to call and didn't.

Each time I heard his voice, smelled his cologne, or heard our song (That darn "*Smooth*," by Santana), some protective body of laws and principles inside the cells of my own body just took over all logic. The fact was, no matter how hard I prayed, my cells were addicted to this guy, and it was going to take me more than just a change of heart to overcome the addiction of him.

♥ It was going to take some real work, emotionally, mentally, and physically. ♥

It actually became an amusing lesson in love boundaries once I got a clue and did some real concentrated emotional healing. Dr. Pat Allen, Ph.D. helped me heal some pretty broken pieces left inside of me from childhood, as well. It wasn't easy, but was definitely worth the effort. I also realized I was going to have to hand those broken pieces over to God, as I had promised. By doing so, God gave me the strength to make some difficult Self♥Love recipes I could have never made on my own.

But I had to continue studying His Word in order to understand how to make those ingredients work, and study I did!

> ♥ Not all of God's ingredients were in line with my convictions at the time of my learning them, but I adopted them as my commitments, and that made all the difference. ♥

I continued to study everything I could get my hands on while holding it up to the light of truth the Bible was speaking to me.

Dr. Crenshaw's book was the single greatest book I have ever read about the influence our sex hormones have over our relationships. It helped me understand the chemical reasons why, and how to literally detoxify myself from Mr. Chemistry's voice, body, pictures, touch, and smell, and why it took me almost six months before I could even begin to think straight. It was that dang DHEA thing!

♥ A Good Case ♥

Chemistry not only influences whom we attract and what we feel, but that it may even tell us whom in particular we want and just how much we want them! There are some great scientifically chemical reasons why a woman should avoid having intimate relations with a man before he gives her his commitment. I'll tell you what; it sure reinforced my trust in the Bible. Yes, I said the Bible.

Dr. Crenshaw makes a good case for why women and men, no matter their age, from a chemical perspective, really should consider some of those Biblical guidelines as more than just rules designed to put the fear of God in you.

My mistake was thinking that after being married for so many years, and now being single again, I didn't really needed to follow those guidelines. I thought they were just silly teenage rules to keep me thinking I'd go straight to hell if I didn't listen to them. Boy, was I wrong. Those guidelines are there for a reason. Like I said, not all of them my convictions, but once I made them my commitment, I understood how powerfully they can work for or against you!

There are chemicals within our bodies (called pheromones) that can actually cause a specific reaction in another person. They even have the power to influence and dictate our behavior without our even realizing it! Some pheromones are as unique to an individual as a fingerprint. Dr. Crenshaw suggests that every individual has what she calls their own "smell-print."

She suggests that each time we move we leave behind a cloud of molecules. Our skin is flooded with these little pheromone molecules, which we slough off at the rate of over one thousand cells per hour! That's a lot of "smell-prints" we are leaving behind, wherever we go.

Some of the pheromones in these smell-prints will affect men and have no affect on women or affect women and not men. They can even affect each person differently, because they act on the brain and nervous system. Although humans have a lot in common, we are all unique. That uniqueness comes from our independent thoughts, motivations, society, stress levels, and childhood brain imprints. It's amazing stuff, this chemistry thing.

I've read that millions of dollars are being spent every day on research to understand and manipulate the general public through pheromone therapies.

Dr. David Berliner, a researcher for Erox Corporation, is concentrating on developing "commercial" pheromones to market to the masses. He has isolated substances from the human skin that behave like sexual pheromones.

> ♥Control the chemistry of the body, and you control the person's choice-making ability, as well. ♥

Crenshaw writes about the managing director of Bodywise, Ltd., a mail order cosmetics company in Australia who sent out one thousand past due bills, half of which were treated with a threatening pig pheromone and half were not. She claims the scented mail ended up paying up by 17% higher than the unscented mail!

Crenshaw also suggests that a woman's sense of smell is more acute than a man's, primarily because of a hormone called estrogen. She says, "Men are not as sensitive to subtle scents, and seem to be able to handle downright rank ones considerably better than women."

Have you ever noticed that a man can sweat and not even know he smells bad? Well, Crenshaw explained this little phenomenon to me. She suggests that it works in a man's favor, as his sweat also contains lots more pheromones. So, if he can stand more of his own stink, and still feel good about himself, Nature's giving him better odds on attracting his chemical match.

Get this, in one study, it was found that by dipping a Q-tip into the male sweat contributed from willing volunteers, and placing the saturated Q-Tip under the nose of irregularly menstruating females three times a day, their menses became regular within just a few months. The fact that a man could have the charisma of a Q-Tip, and, as long as you are in regular contact with his sweat, your body will respond to him kind of makes me want to rethink the whole sweaty nightclub scene!

♥ Pheromones ♥

Well, since we can't smell a pheromone like we can a scent, we have to rely on our nervous system to respond emotionally or physically, without any conscious realization of what's going on. This is assuming your nervous system isn't already working overtime with your life's other issues!

It made me wonder what other aspects of my chemistry I was responding to unknowingly, especially when I put myself in unnecessary situations. Perhaps it did make sense to go back to some of those old rules mom and grandma used to preach about. It's chemical warfare out there, and after reading up on the subject I realized I had placed myself in the middle of a battle!

I suspect that the influences of these chemical stimulations on my feelings and my behavior were more powerful than we can currently pinpoint with our scientific minds. In my case, take the hot Summer nights, fill them with Nature's energy, mix in a little toxic Self♥Love-potion, a compulsive addiction to appeasement, throw in a little chemical bondage between two people in the heat of Summer, and guess what:

> ♥You have the perfect recipe for disaster! Or, in my case, a lesson in love on a road trip with God.♥

♥The Earlier Question♥

So, going back to the earlier question, why did I keep letting the same guy teach me the same lesson over and over again? Why did I keep making the same mistakes?

I surmised from reading Crenshaw's book that it had an awful lot to do with chemistry. In addition, I was looking in the wrong place for true love, altogether.

It was time to heal my broken pieces. It was time to hand over my psychological, emotional, physical, and Spiritual broken pieces to God and let Him lead me out of this mess I had gotten my life into.

I finally realized that Mr. Chemistry and I really had nothing else going on between us besides our chemistry and the season. I was in love with a seasonal serial monogamist! Yup, that's what I called him. Happy and available for a serious relationship for two to three months, then on to the next season. I knew the signs pretty well.

As I improved in my ability to *take a "moment" with God* in between contacts with this walking hormone magnet who owned my chemistry, I began to see the healing lesson revealing itself. It became clearer to me why some relationships made it through all four of Nature's seasons (a lifetime of seasons in some cases), while others only made it through a season or two, with seemingly hallucinogenic highs and potentially volatile lows, like mine.

"Next Summer would be different," I declared, as I continued to learn.

Even though I was still clutching to the hope that eventually Mr. Chemistry might still come around, I decided to escape to Cabo San Lucas, Mexico, with my girlfriends, when what, to my wondering eyes, should appear? The same man, with a different face, dancing and sweating in the hot Summer nightclub, away from reality and in the light of a full Summer's moon.

> ♥ Another irresistible chemical hormone magnet of men, who also believed he could just pick me up and take me wherever he wanted me to go? I Don't Think So! ♥

I had learnt the red flags well by now and I was able to resist my own chemistry by logically (and prayerfully) acknowledging the potential hazard standing there in front of me in that hot and sweaty club.

"It ain't going to be that effortless, mister," I said, purposefully. At least I was *determined* not to make it easy for him. Once he found out that we only lived a few miles from each other back in California he persisted until I finally accepted a lunch date. I had thrown his business card away three times by then!

He knew his body had met its chemical match, too. But the key was, because I recognized the signs early on, I was able to avoid another chemical addiction. I was able to discern my way through the relationship in a considerably healthier manner than the Summer relationship I'd had before. As a matter of fact, we are still great friends to this day.

♥Short vs. Long-Term Relationships♥

I've become quite competent at identifying the potential for short-term and long-term relationships. Short-term, often chemically explosive relationships appear to throw caution to the wind and rely heavily on thermodynamics and chance; in other words, just letting Nature take its course without conscious thought to the outcome of those choices.

I see them more often during the Spring and Summer months, but certainly they can happen any time of year when you meet your chemical match. There is not a lot of logic associated with many of the actions displayed in a short-term relationship, and the common goal is usually instant gratification. These encounters are better described as "situations," rather than relationships. They tend to end as quickly, and sometimes as dramatically, as they got started, leaving nothing but burnt embers in their wake.

> ♥Then there are the long-term potential relationships.
> They are the ones that appear to be more purpose driven and
> Spirit based. ♥

The long-term potentials that can avoid the pitFalls of early chemical ambush generally demonstrate common goals and philosophies within their structures. They tend to be made up of two individuals who each contribute their unique gifts and strengths to lift the other up, without considering themselves any less by doing so.

Remember that list I had created earlier? The one of the perfect man? I was considering all the things that were missing from that list. When I asked God to lead me to the man who held me in chemical bondage for over a year, I didn't realize how important those missing trivialities are. A man's character, loyalty, and trust are distinct parts of the foundational make up of a long-term (chemically-charged or not) relationship. The things I had on my list were "great catch potential" qualities, which no woman should feel uncomfortable asking from God. But focusing only on these things can be as illusory as chemistry, if it's all he's got going for him.

Once I asked myself, how I would feel, or what I would think of Mr. Chemistry if he lost his financial security, dressed differently, was unable to take me to the fun places he took me, drove a different car, etc. What would be leftover that I would find attractive?

Was I considering how wonderful he was for other women to look at, thus elevating him so much that I couldn't see my own values and strengths when I stood next to him? I had done that in my marriage, so perhaps I was doing it again.

A few insights my grandma shared with me came to mind,

> ♥ If he can't take care of you any better than you can take care of yourself, you're wasting your time, and I ain't just talking about money, honey! ♥

Now, lest your brain goes right into the gutter on that statement, Grandma wasn't talking about sex. What she was referring to is that it's normal and healthy for a woman to look for the alpha-male (a man a little higher up the ladder, or at least on the same rung as she is) but what's most important is a man's level of character: his level of integrity, loyalty, and trustworthiness.

Grandma would wisely and softly remind me. "Once a man has reached his full potential, whether you helped him get there or not, you better be able to trust what he is going to do from then on. Things like Spirituality and faith help strengthen the fabric of a man's character."

Grandma was a sensible old woman.

In long-term (life-time) relationships, I saw common goals, philosophies, emotional maturity, stability, consistency, and realistic expectations of one another. It takes character and Spiritual maturity, on both parts, to really pull it off, I think.

Seasonal serial monogamy, however, can have all the flavor and feeling of a long-term relationship, but will only last only for three to four months, and then end, leaving oneself to be available (with the same potential on display), for the next chemical victim. I suppose it's not necessarily a bad thing, if you're aware and up front about the fact that you don't want a permanent or long-term relationship. But it can be devastating if you don't know you're doing it, or having it done to you.

The phrase "fear of intimacy" comes to mind, and that kind of fear will always lead to the end of a relationship with gut-wrenching sobs.

> ♥ Speaking from experience, it's the kind of sobbing where you're left clutching your knees to your chest, and your insides feel like they are going to come up and out through your mouth. ♥

But, on the other hand, they can be quite exciting and turn out to be the "times of your life" kind of adventures. With a carefree attitude, they can be quite painless, unless of course, it's the end of the season, and you happened to be really in love with that (now dying) seasonal flower! I tried to explain this theory to my girlfriend using the following garden metaphor.

♥ Seasonal Flower Garden of Love ♥

In any garden, some blossoms will last longer than others, depending on the kind of blossoms you pick and the season in which you pick it. Once the season begins to change, if the roots of the plant you're picking your blossoms from are unable to grow deep enough beneath the soil, the plant is unable to withstand the elements and the blossoms stop looking so attractive.

When the libidinous nutrients of the flower bed are consumed too quickly, (chemical passion), they leave the soil (self-esteem), depleted, and the entire plant (excitement of the relationship) withers and dies. That's when the weeds (arguments, avoidance behavior), begin to choke the very life out of any further potential the plant may have had (And you can forget about it producing any more blossoms, too!) Since Mother Nature never wastes her energy, she just sends in the parasites to clean up the mess and re-nourish the soil for the next season of plants. We call that "lessons!"

Perennial plants (the year round, long-term kind), tend to grow in a deep-rooted environment and will bloom year after year. Generally this plant is found within a prayerfully well thought-out, well-maintained, and regularly replenished garden. The weeds are faithfully and perpetually being pulled, allowing the roots of that relationship to grow deeper with each season. Though the blossoms may still come forward abundantly during one or two seasons, the plant is constantly being nourished, with Self♥Love Potions added to the soil, and will always maintain its green luster, even after the blooms fade from sight.

Ask any gardener and they can tell you, it is absolutely impossible to grow a garden full of beautiful flowers simply by pulling weeds. Duhhh! So no matter how much Mother Nature has nourished the soil, you absolutely can not have a thriving plant, nor a blossom for that matter, until you get you a little something to start with first. You know, a seed, a root, a cutting (even a weed can turn to a bloom!). And guess what?

Sometimes chemistry may just be that little seedling that gets you started. So it's not always a bad thing to be chemically crazy about your partner.

The Self♥Love lesson here is to be discerning about the environment in which you choose to plant and grow your seeds, and know what kind of plant you're trying to get to bloom. Is it a weed, a perennial or an evergreen?

There were many a night I spent bent on my knees, clutching an empty flower vase, like a small child holding its pacifier, trying to figure out how come the neighbor had a garden so full of color, while all I had was a wilted, dying plant, and I was putting way more time into my garden then she was!

I'd do a rain dance, throw a fit, kill a bug or two, and plead with God not to let me live out the rest of my life without a deep-rooted connection. It's not that I didn't have other plants that wanted to bloom in my garden; it's just that I wanted to save the wilted dying ones by pouring chemical fertilizer over the dead leaves on a hot Summer day. I didn't even know that I was killing every thing else in my garden by focusing all my energy on performing a miracle to save the dying weed!

I don't know about you, but I just hate the feeling of rejection, even from a "dead" plant. I'm just not good at it, but as I watched Mother Nature send her parasites in on a feeding frenzy, devouring every resemblance of what was once a blossoming Summer wildflower, I realized there was nothing I could do to make that plant bloom again. Its season was over; it had served its purpose, and it was time to get a wiser gardener than me: God.

♥ Returning to the Ride ♥

With all my strength and newfound tools of information, I asked myself again, *What part of me still needs to feel not good enough? What part of me needs to prove how very special I am by accomplishing the impossible fairy tale with a man incapable of being a prince?*

And the answer came from the warm Summer wind, "The broken pieces of your heart, my dear,"

It was time to serve myself the truth. I got down on my knees and offered God my broken pieces, while I could still think straight.

I was tired of carrying all those broken pieces around with me, anyway. Each time someone would extend their hand to me, I'd would always drop a piece or two on the ground, and I would be the one stepping all over it, while trying to pick it back up. So, the answer to the question, "What part of me still needs this lesson?" NONE!

"Go home and pack your things, My little angel," God's voice sang to me. "I'll be 'round to get you later on this evening. You are ready for the rest of your road trip, aren't you?" He said, pausing for emphasis.

I went straight home. I lit a pink candle, put on some peppermint essential oil, played Santana at full volume and reached up to remove the diamond earrings my heart's captor had placed in my ears that hot Summer past. He must have sensed the closure on an ethereal level somehow, because at that very moment, I heard the phone ring. It was him! All this time, and now he calls?

Fortunately I allowed the answering machine to pick up the message as he left his invitation to "get together."

Why was he calling? I thought to myself as I turned down the music.

I must have replayed his message a dozen times, hoping to hear something more than just the words. Then it hit me like a ton of bricks: *Why would I even be thinking about letting my heart go there again with him?*

That was it! I wasn't going to choose that for my life anymore. I was finally strong enough to see him in a different light. He hadn't changed—I had. He was behaving just as he always had. He wasn't doing anything new or wrong, that's just really who he was. So in the end, the only thing that was going to make a difference was me.

With that, I hit the triangular shaped button on the center of the answering machine, that read "Erase." I sashayed my way back into the living room and blasted Santana's *Smooth* loud enough for the entire neighborhood to hear.

"…make it real, or just forget about it…!" I sang, dancing around the room.

Just then, God showed up, and walked right over to the stereo, stopping the music altogether.

"It's about time you got it! I was getting sick of hearing that song, anyway!" He said, jokingly. "For the rest of your road trip, there is going to be more peace and quiet. I want you to hear yourself think, and understand what it is you are feeling, and when you're ready, I want you to dance and sing to the music of your heart, understand?" He stated more than He asked.

God has helped me laugh at myself more times than I care to mention. With God leading the way, I've learned that

> ♥ True love is not something I get from someone else; it is something I had to fill myself with first. ♥

I had been confusing romantic love with Self ♥ Love, man after perfect man, because I had more fear than Self ♥ Love in me when I started this road trip. There was little room to accept another's offerings, no matter how much I wanted them. I really didn't understand what Self ♥ Love was until God let me learn through the lessons of my Mr. Chemistry and my Mr. Right NOWs. Those poor guys. I mean they can only be expected to try so hard, for so long, before eventually one of us would give up saying, "I'm done. I can't make you happy." And you know what? We were right. We can't make other people happy. That's something we have to do for ourselves.

> ♥Learning how to make myself happy was the first of many powerful Self♥Love lessons that followed. ♥

♥Unhealed Hell♥

Experiencing the painful truth that there was no man on this earth that would ever feel like a success in my presence, as long as I kept the broken pieces of my heart unhealed and hidden inside of me, was a lesson worth learning.

Oh, the hell I've put some men through. But handing over the broken pieces of our hearts is a choice that initiates consequences each of us must experience for ourselves. It took me a while to even locate some of those broken pieces, because I had so successfully hidden them so deep inside. God has been exquisitely graceful at teaching me how to find, and hand over those pieces to Him.

With a twinge of embarrassment and affection, I've come to discern that if a man feels like a failure in my presence, he is innately programmed to wave and point his finger about, shouting something like, "I will not be forgotten, abandoned, or ignored!" and expect little more in those moments than for me to simply smile back at him, confidently, with adoration and appreciation, as if I should have known as much in the first place! My view of this lesson is far grander today in comparison to the mere snapshot I had of it at the beginning of my road trip.

There were lots of lessons in love I had to learn. Each time I felt romantically ambushed, I'd turn to God with my tear-filled, questioning eyes, trying to convince Him that I felt love's lessons were eventually going to turn me into a permanently disheartened creature! I recall the time I mustered my courage up enough to actually demand that God reveal His hidden agenda for my heart! Oh, so many times I wanted to just get right out of that limo and walk back home because I knew it was my free will to be there in the first place. I could have chosen to quit at any time, but I am wiser for the investment of my time and patience.

When God finally did reply, His words were powerful and forthright.

"I have no hidden agenda to mire you in, or romantically ambush you with. I expose Me, the Truth, as often as I can to you, not to evoke more than you are willing to give or learn. I do not ask, nor do I expect. You are empowered by your own choosing. I simply drive the car toward revealing your true nature. And, if you're tired of feeling like you are just driving around in circles, why don't you just stop trying to drive, and just sit there and paint your toenails for a while, hmmmm? I do know where I've got to get you"

You'd think I'd have learned to just sit back and do as I was told, but nooooo. In my impatience, every time God got out of the car to stretch His legs, I'd jump right into the driver's seat again and try to take control.

It's human nature to do so, I guess. But one thing I did learn: God will not be rushed any more than Mother Nature will. Every time I tried to sneak up in the front seat of that big old limo and drive off, before I even knew where I was going—yeah, you guessed it—I'd get lost again. God was so patient with me, though. He'd just wait for me to turn the car around and invite Him back in. He always knew I would find my way back to Him, so He would just stand there and wait for me to bring His car back to Him.

I asked Him why He was never mad that I left Him like that, and how come He was always so sure I would come back again? He just smiled and said,

"It's like walking toward an electric door; I know you're coming, and I automatically open up for you." Then He added, "And I always will."

I know the price for wisdom is often suffering, and God would tell me that it was because I honestly sought His wisdom that He could use that suffering to help me heal. My seeking also empowered Him to help me.

"I delight in our time together, My dear. In My accepting way, I see any time you take to share with Me as a measure of your love. I accept these moments as your gifts of affection. I can see the truth and the struggles that lie buried within the broken pieces of your heart. One day you'll realize I am not here to capture or obligate you, and you'll begin to consider Me a more trusted companion, too. That's when I become the driver of the vehicle of true love in your life. Isn't that what you asked for in the first place?" He would say, intent on His composure, but revealing His true vulnerability in loving me so.

I nodded my head, "Yes."

In return He'd cradle my chin in His mighty right hand and said, "Ah, but first come the lessons that reveal Truth. Now move over and study this map for Me, and when you think you're willing to follow it, I'll feel much better about letting you drive again."

Then He flashed me that peaceful look and reassured me that eventually I would get there.

> ♥ Grace, and all its underlying uniqueness, was revealed to me in those moments. ♥

I learned a great deal about fear on those days, and how it can mess with God in my head. I felt more empowered each time I returned to Him. Eventually, I was able to just simply accept His strength and allow that energy to move through me, as I handled the difficult situations of my life.

God made it clear beyond words that I didn't know as much as I thought I did, but that He would always be by my side, though every season of my life.

> ♥ Even healers need healing, I guess. ♥

Chapter Six

Chapter Six

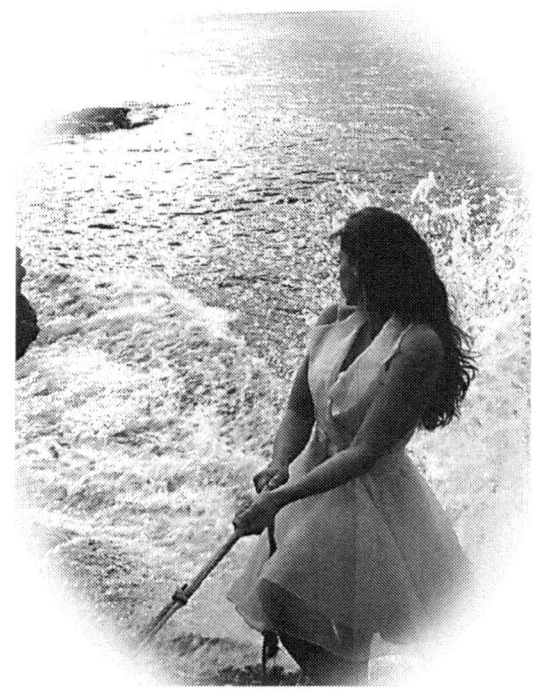

♥ *A Loving Voice*

You are safe. I have offered my life up to the Lord as an empty vessel through which He may Love you, and my commitment is to my last breath.

♥Whispers of Winter's Wisdom

♥Ocean "Moments" ♥

Sometimes, in the early morning hours, when no else is around, I like to walk down to the beach where I am able to take in Nature's refreshing perspective of my life. It's there that I give myself a good dose of faith-filled conversations with God. As a rule, I tend to get quite deep and philosophical during these early morning consultations, especially during Winter's dialogues. I let my mind, thoughts, feelings and heart just merge and become one with the abandoned sands.

As I watch the moon give way to the sunrise, and the beach give way to the rising tide, I'll pick up a stone and toss it across a tide pool. The beach of Winter is the perfect place for me to take a moment to reset and listen to my inner voice. My soul knows I crave more than just the formal subduing of Winter. You know, like the traditional baking of cookies and wrapping of presents. Then there is my Winter body...and my body knows it's going to take more than an extra spin class to balance out my emotions.

During this cooling time of year, my soul considers itself more than just a helping hand, when it comes to connecting my body, mind, and inner communication with Winter's message. The beach seems to be the perfect place for me to just sit and listen to myself think. It's where I can and really hear what it is I'm feeling.

A few days ago, as I was sitting there on the beach, breathing in and allowing my body chemistry to relax to the rhythms of the ocean. I thought I heard someone whispering, but, when I looked around, there was nothing there but the tide pools and me. I closed my eyes again, and, as soon as I did, I heard the words:

Tests of Faith.

Opening my eyes and seeing that there was still no one there, I kind of got goose bumps, but then brushed it off to too much caffeine before my morning walk. I began, once again, to give in to the awesome feeling of being connected to the oceans rhythms.

Test of Faith. Tests of…

Trying to ignore the distracting sound of someone's voice, I just concentrated harder on the melodic sound of my environment.

Test of Faith!

I heard again louder and louder until finally the sound broke through my ability to concentrate, and, a little more than irritated, I opened my eyes. Fully expecting to see someone standing right next to me I grumbled,

"That is really rude! Can't you see I'm trying to have a "moment" here?!?"

Realizing there was still no one standing there, and now feeling a little foolish, I rose to my feet and made my way closer to where I thought I heard the voice coming from. Looking up I saw two love birds cozied up together inside a shaded cavern. All around me were God's creatures, scurrying and oblivious to my existence. Overhead were seagulls and clouds gliding carelessly though the blue morning sky. The scent of the ocean's golden gifts advancing and retreating along the foamy current drew my attention toward her as I placed my feet within a tide pool of water.

Ahhh, so that's what's making that sound, I said to myself, as I watched the ocean's tide pull cords of seaweed along the mossy rocks. She spoke in an almost inaudible voice, yet one that only my intuition would be able to decipher.

"Okay," I said taking a seat beside the moving seabed. "I'll play; what do you have to say to me this morning?" half looking over my shoulder to see if anyone was going to catch me talking to a bunch of seaweed.

"Tests of Faith," the seaweed sang.

Sitting there, alone with my thoughts, God, and Nature, it was hard to pinpoint just who was really speaking to whom. Letting go further of my conscious understanding of the words, I asked the question,

"Okay, testing faith or faith testing, what exactly is are you trying to say to me?

The water retreated silently, perhaps to gather an answer, then play-fully splashed forward her response,

"Did you know that test of Faith, when offered by God, is far differ-ent than you testing your faith based on God's response to you?"

"Hmmm," I said sticking my finger into the cool tide pool just in time to touch the tail of a curious fish.

"So you're suggesting, what? I am testing God or God is testing me right now?" I asked while my hand continued to chase the fish about the mossy plants.

"The answer is yes; there is a test of Faith currently going on in your life. The question is: Are you going to test your own faith by demanding God respond to your specific wishes, or are you going to hold onto your faith in Him, while He demonstrates to you how peaceful your life can be by the realizing the power of having faith in Him," the seabed spoke.

"Ok, now wait a minute. Just because I expect God to answer my prayers doesn't mean I'm testing my faith, does it?" I said, pulling my hand from the water and wiping the wetness onto my shirt.

"Only when your trust in God is contingent upon God's specific response to your demands, my little starfish!" Then the water went silent.

"So you're suggesting that I may be in the midst of a test, and the only way to be sure I am not testing my own faith is to seek God's guidance and wisdom, and then trust God, and not myself, no matter what it feels like at that moment. Right?" I asked, noticing the morning sunrise announcing her arrival with a brilliant display of reflective sparkle that danced off the ocean's waves.

"If you find yourself in a difficult situation and demand God get you out of it, God may or may not grant your request, but His silence does not mean He is not with you during your struggles, or that your faith in Him has been in vain. You understand that, right?" the seabed offered, as she showered forth in foaming reverberation.

Looking out over the ocean I countered, "So you're saying that when I demand God answer me, and He doesn't answer me the way I want Him to, I should not get mad at God. Rather, I should just trust that God can always hear me but, because of my own free will, I may have freely made a choice that put me in the middle of an uncomfortable situation, and God is allowing me to struggle for a reason, if He doesn't answer my SPECIFIC prayer exactly the way I pray it. Right?" I said, waiving my finger at the misty ocean air and then tossing a pebble across the glistening pools, pausing provokingly for the answer.

The rippling tide responded, "If you keep your eyes focused on the bigger picture of God's plan for your life, even when you can't see or understand it at the time, you won't become bitter toward God for the suffering, and, in a sense, you will be letting God heal you, strengthen you, and, in turn, use the lessons of your tender failures to heal others in the same situations, later," the ocean added, with a undulating splash for emphasis.

Supervising a crab scuttling across the pointed rocks, I measured the ocean's declaration by drawing in a deep and comforting chestful of ocean air. This was a familiar message. I had read it somewhere before. Feeling the cool mist expanding in my lungs, I eventually returned the air to its lender and replied,

"Ok, this is getting a little deep, but I'll go with it just for another minute. Am I to believe that the painful situations in my life are actually God's will for my life, if I've prayed before hand and things still turn out bad?" I said, crossing my arms over my chest.

"Because if that's what you're suggesting, I'm not so sure I buy into that theory. Why would a loving God want me to feel pain? Any kind of pain? And I certainly can't see how my struggles could possibly be used to heal someone else's hurts? That just doesn't make any sense," I stated, turning my face away from the water's edge, and expressing, with body language more than words, that I was beginning to tire of this game the ocean tides were playing with my thoughts.

The ocean began, pulling in her breath,

"Isn't it true that you are more willing to change when something hurts you, than when everything is going along just great in your life?" the ocean questioned, continuing to draw in smoothly as if calculating the timing of her retort.

"When you gave your life over to God, you gave your life over in faith. GOD'S tests of Faith are designed to help you grow, and if He uses pain to get your attention, your willingness to trust God through these tests becomes more important then the answers as to why He is not getting you out of that pain or why you have pain in the first place!" the ocean blared with a persuasive shower of cool water powerful enough to cause me to uncross my arms.

Wiping the water from my face and turning my attention toward the sound of burbling water that was now draining from the soaked rocks beds overhead, I countered,

"Well, I believe that God delights in me being happy no matter what you say, and I still can't see how me having pain in my life could possibly serve God's will. I'm not asking for it, and He can't possibly believe I need any more of it," feeling like a defiant little mermaid as I watched the water cascade down the Cliffside.

"Oh, my…you are a precocious little starfish, aren't you! I can see you are going to require some convincing," the sea announced, as the trickles sang in unison, racing toward the lower pools in a flamboyant display of overflow.

"It would do you good to simply accept the discomforts in your life as part of your life's path," the ocean wailed, as she thundered into the rocky cliffs with a demonstration of her force so expressive, I could distinguish the lingering vibrations throughout the tide pools for several moments.

"The question is: Are you going to do something good with the lessons of that pain, or let the lessons be wasted on you?"

"Good gosh!" I said, wiping the foam from my face and watching the water drip down the front of my shirt. Noticing a crab that had been shaken from its hiding place, I eagerly scooped it up. After allowing a few more moments to pass without saying anything, I finally responded.

"Well, I just don't see the need to sit here contemplating all the why's of the worst and most painful moments in my life. Next thing I know, you're going to be telling me to write it all down, and share these moments with the whole wide world, like that's going to somehow help someone!"

The crab quickly jumped from my hand and escaped toward the safety of another hidden cavern. With a surprised giggle I continued, "I am sure the loving God I know gave me a brain so I could use it to think my way through any situation, and the smarter I get, the less pain I'll have in my life." Continuing to pursue the crab, "I am not going to make the same mistakes I did before. And as far as anyone else learning from my mistakes, well, I've learned my lessons and I think that's all that's important, Mr. Seabed, regardless of who is testing whom," I continued as the crab disappeared from view.

Pausing briefly, the ocean once again withdrew from the tide pool.

"You don't have to be perfect to help someone else; you just have to be one step ahead of them to offer them a hand forward. It's time you learned that lesson, and learned how to stay out of trouble while you help others with what you've experienced in your own life, little one," she whispered, as she retreated from the cliff.

"Oh, sure, now you back down," I said standing erect and placing my hands upon my hips.

"So where ya going?" I yelled tauntingly.

"What, you don't want to play anymore because I made a good case for myself, hmmmm?" I asserted, believing the ocean feared the boldness of my truths by its retreat.

Just then, I felt a gust of wind blow up against my back so strongly that it caused me to reconsider my footing on the cliff's edge. I took a step back and turned my face into the insistent wind.

"That attitude is the very thing that gets you into most of the painful situations in your life, my child. Did you ever stop to think that some of your problems really have nothing to do with you, but have everything to do with helping other people?" the wind howled, cautiously pushing at my chest. The voice had a very familiar tone to it.

"God, is that you?" I considered in my thoughts.

"When you invited Me into your life, you offered Me your life to use as "I" see fit. By following Me during the most painful situations of your life, you're allowing Me to use you as an encouragement to others. Do not be so quick to forget the lessons each pain has taught you. True, it is good to focus on those things that are right and true, light and beautiful. However, My desire for you is for you to share your failures, faults, frustrations, fears, and feelings with those who may need your experience with such matters. I will always comfort you in your troubles, so that you can offer that same comfort to others when they are in trouble. If you shared only from your strengths, it would be too easy for others to discount your triumphs, writing them off to just being lucky or simply being born that way. That is not My intent for your life's painful experiences, My child. Everyone will have disappointments in their lives, just like you, but your faith is what gives you hope, and hope gives the world eyes to see My working all things together for the good of those who desire My will for their lives."

I stood there for what seemed like hours but could not have been more than a few seconds. Rushes of emotions filled me as I steadied myself against the winds that surrounded me. Lowering my eyes I whispered under my breath,

"All I was saying is that I didn't really want to sit around here revisiting all my mistakes," muttering and pushing up against the tip of a black and white shell with the rubber-soled portion of my sandals.

"How come you can't just talk to me like a regular person, so I understand more clearly what you're trying to say? Is that my test? Am I supposed to figure out how to use my past hurts to help others?" I pouted, still grumbling under my breath.

I grabbed hold of a protruding rock to steady myself as I lowered my body below the sweeping progress of the gusting wind and continued with my thoughts.

The sound of another thunderous boom caused me to raise an eyebrow. Nestling further inside the gutted cavern of the cliffside, I stuck my finger into the mouth of an anemone. "Tickle…tickle…tickle," I giggled, as the multi-colored tentacles suckled on my hand. The ocean rushed up and over the hallowed rock and plunged into the pools in front of me with a mighty force. As quickly as the wave lunged forward, she fell back, leaving endless steaming children chasing after her.

Hoping that boom was that last of the ocean's exclamation points to her earlier statements, I brushed the sand from my legs and peeked out across the overhang toward the ocean, hoping to discover a more calming tone. Rising to my feet I offered,

"Um, listen, just because I don't understand why or how doesn't mean I can't at least try to figure something out, Ck? Even if I am gonna sound like a nut-case when I try to explain all this to someone, one day."

Taking the opportunity to escape from the ocean's reach, I began jumping and leaping over tide pools. Behind me, I heard the sound of a powerful surge of rushing water. The reality of the impending danger that was gathering strength before me, and the magnitude of what was happening began to settle in.

♥The Beginning♥

Earlier that morning I had been walking along the beach, as I always do. I came to the point in the shoreline where I couldn't walk any farther, because the rocky cliff protrudes out into the ocean. It was a low tide, and the water had receded back far enough to expose the remnants of a tattered rope that had been secured around a large boulder. I had considered climbing over that boulder a few days earlier, but was cautioned to retreat by a climber returning from the other side.

"The tide is shifting, and it's too dangerous, right now," he said.

I asked him what was on the other side, and he told me,

"It's where Mother Nature stands naked."

Smiling with intrigue I added, "And I bet it's so beautiful, because not many people know it's there, huh?"

"Or make it that far. Even if you do make it that far, Nature won't let you stay too long, because of the rapid tide changes in the cove, so you be careful if you ever go it on your own, Okay?" he cautioned.

So I acquiesced on that morning. However, today, on this particular sunrise, there, in the presence of a low tide and a full moon in the morning mist, that rope was fully exposed, and was calling my name.

I began to climb the jagged pathway, keeping in mind the promised reward on the other side. As I risked getting swept off of the slippery boulders and thrown up against the rocky shoreline by a crashing wave,

I felt my heart skip a beat. Finally reaching the rope, I grabbed hold of one of the slipknots someone had made to aid the climber's grip. I used them to help me pull myself up and over what was the largest rock barrier between me and the sandy lagoon on the other side.

Pulling myself across the slippery, jagged edges, I heard someone yell from the beach,

"If you're not sure you can time your return before the tide comes up, turn back now, because once you're on the other side of that cliff, there is no way out but the way you go in".

"Thanks," I shouted back with a wave that almost caused me to lose my footing and let go of the rope completely. Fortunately I had a firm grasp with my other hand and only slipped a few inches down the razor sharp pathway. As I pulled myself up and over the rock, Nature saluted my courage with one of the most beautiful sights imaginable.

Ignoring the throbbing sensation in my leg, I continued on until I finally made my way down into the lagoon. I felt validated and insignificant, both at the same time. Nature was speaking to the most primal parts of my being. My connection to this massive body of energy was without words, without conscious thought; without articulable feelings, yet, she was communication with all of these senses at once.

"Visual proof that God exists," Nature spoke to me, without using words.

Wow," I thought, "*most people probably never get this far.*

I reached down to slow the bleeding from my leg and silently hoped I had some calendula and comfrey back home to pack on my leg to help prevent any infection.

Making my way down to the sandy white lagoon, I drank in the purity of God's creations, all scurrying about. Moving closer to a tide pool to splash the cooling fluid over my abraded skin, I let my mind race with my thoughts, out over the rippling currents. As I became absorbed in the moon giving way to the morning sun, the tides began to speak to me: "Tests of Faith"…and so the conversation began.

Now, no longer deep in thought and introspection, my mind was filling with alarm. Seeing the waves building in the distance I raced back toward the shelter of the cavern I had just emerged from. I could feel the throbbing in my leg return. Blood began to trickle down my leg and mix with the rising tide as my heart began to race from adrenaline.

Looking at my watch, I realized I had been there for hours, and somehow the time had gotten way from me. What's more, Nature had given me plenty of warning of her shifting tides, but I wasn't even paying attention. The retreating lagoons, the winds, the crashing waves— God wasn't scolding me after all, He was just telling me He didn't want me in that lagoon any longer.

How many other messages had I prayed for, only to confuse the true meaning of the answers? How many other times in my life did I mistake God's "not nows" "for nos?" I felt like Elijah when he was angry with God for drying up the riverbed. Elijah asked God why He was so angry with him, and what he could have done to deserve such punishment. God's reply, in essence, was, "I'm not mad at you, Elijah. I just don't want you here anymore."

And so it goes with following God's will over following my own! I got the lesson the ocean was trying to deliver.

With the water now rising above my ankles, I could feel my heart competing with my mind for clarity.

Well, so much for the 'predictable' rising tide, I thought, realizing I had gotten myself stuck in a pretty serious situation.

Listening for the ocean to steady herself, in between the heaving of thousands of gallons of water that she was slamming into the rocks and spraying over my head, I nestled as deep as I could into the side of the bluff. Hearing the ocean retreat to gather her strength, I peeked around the cavern to see how far I would have to run in between sets. I had to reach the large boulder in the cliff's edge before the next large wave, and make my way up to that rope, in order to return to the civilized side of the beach.

As I looked ahead, I was shocked to find that boulder was barely peeking at me, from in between very large sets of forcefully crashing waves. Seeing as how that was my only way out of the lagoon, which was also about to be re consumed by the rising tides, I didn't have a choice but to start running, NOW!

"Talk about testing your faith; I suppose you're going to tell me that God is going to use this little experience for good somehow!" I shouted as I ran from one rocky cavern to the next, hoping not to get caught off guard by the booming tide.

Feeling the pain in my leg growing more noticeable with each step, I said out loud, "How do I get myself into these messes?"

Stopping only long enough to catch my breath I continued ranting, "Why did God have to show me that dang rope in the first place?"

"To see the rope is one thing. You chose to grab hold of it!" the ocean taunted. "You had to calculate the risk, ignore the warnings of those who have come before you. Even with a wounded leg, you still chose to use what other physical strengths you had, to pull yourself up and over the jagged edges of the cliff. Once at the top you saw the beauty of the lagoon. You could have been satisfied and turned back. You didn't. You chose to go forward and climb down into the lagoon. You chose to listen for and then listen to the message being delivered to you now. You are always being offered the choices, but you are the one doing the choosing, little starfish," the ocean shouted, with a massive discharge of water that sounded like a thousand-urchin choir.

Oh great insight, I shouted to myself, realizing I was now yelling in an audible voice at the ocean.

"Can't you make my lessons any more clear than these dim-witted metaphors you keep talking in?" I yelled, as I took advantage of the ocean's calmness and applied more pressure to my bleeding leg.

"Why don't you try a metaphor yourself, little starfish, and I'll give you a few moments to gather your strength before you have to run for the boulder with the rope," the ocean responded in her silence.

Weighing my options, and realizing I didn't have many, nor did I have too far to go before I reached the foot of the pathway leading to the rope, I accepted the offer and tended my wound.

"Okay, there are people in this world that come to the cliffs of life far more prepared than me, and hundreds of others, just like me, that are taking the journey one step and one lesson at a time. How's that?" I asked, fully expecting a discernible reply.

"Good, keep going," the ocean encouraged, as she too rested to catch her breath.

"Okay, look, if God would have me use my life's pain to provide a little advice that won't confuse, discourage or lead others to withdraw from their lives' purpose, then I guess that wouldn't be so bad," I said, beginning to move, once again, toward the rope. "People only get the lessons of their lives when they're ready to hear the words, so maybe my stories can make a difference, somehow,"

Finally reaching the pathway that led up the pebble strewn cliff, I began the climb. I continued the conversation with myself, out loud, as if doing so would somehow stop the fear of drowning that was beginning to take over my rational thinking altogether. Grabbing and clawing at the moisture covered rocks, I began pulling myself up with sheer determination.

"Okay, what is the lesson? I know that I got over here because I chose to come," I said, as I continued to pull myself along the cliff, stopping only long enough to avoid being hit by the after-splash of another thunderous wave. "And though I don't regret one moment of sitting in that lagoon, I do regret not paying attention to Nature's reminder that it was time for me to leave." I whined, as yet another wave approached.

Then I heard my attempt at a metaphor turn into a real live prayer, "Lord, please don't let me die like this! It's not my time to die yet. I have so much to write about, and I promise I will write out the stories of my healed hurts, if it will serve Your will for my life. But I can't do that if I'm floating out to sea as shark bait, now, can I? So, could you please help me get out of here, and do it quickly?" I said, finally reaching the rope.

Suspended in mid-air by a tenuous grip on the old and fraying rope, I attempted to time my descent to the safe side of the boulder between the intermittent fury of the crashing waves. Less than secure, with my footing on the blind, downside of a mossy, urchin-covered rock, I just hung there for a moment, hoping God was going to hear my prayer and wondering if there was really any way for me to make it out of there on my own.

Hanging there, I wondered, *If I do make it out, how will I know if it was, indeed, God helping me find my footing and holding back the waves, so I could climb down the rock safely, or if it was my own strength? Or, is there really no way to tell? What was I really doing there in the first place? It's not like God came right out and told me to go climb into that lagoon. It was my choice to do the climbing. Maybe God even tried to warn me not to go in, by causing the injuries to my leg. So, really,* I thought, *He has no responsibility to answer my prayers to get me out.*

Then again, maybe He did inspire me to climb into that lagoon, so I could hear this message and do His will, with what I take away from this experience. If I truly believe God is with me no matter where I go, and I am truly seeking His will for my life, then He can take me anywhere He wants me to go, as well as carry me through any situation. And I can trust that, no matter the outcome of this, or any situation in my life, He is going to use it for good, somehow, and all I have to do is hang in there (literally), and trust Him.

"But, what if you don't get out alive? Then what purpose did it serve to listen to the message in the first place?" challenged the sea, eaves-dropping on my thoughts.

"In that case, it would be the right information, too late! I guess the choice is really up to me, either way," I shouted back, with gathering determination that such would not be the case.

As I hung there, the waves crashing harder and harder against my back, pulling me left and right, away from the rock, I realized that the only thing keeping me from becoming shark bait was my grip on that tattered old rope. The inner and outer aspects of my worlds began to merge. Closing my eyes, I began to listen for the clues that Nature was offering me. In between sets of forceful waves, there was a calming. I let my thinking mind withdraw from the lead, and let my inner senses find the memory of where to place my foot on the downside of the rocky cliff.

My faith is like this rope, I said to myself, continuing the dialogue, *I trust God is here with me and, no matter what, today is not my day to die. I am going to hold on to this rope and my faith. The waves can come crashing but I will not let go.*

My faith allowed my courage to emerge, and the pain in my leg subsided. My inner senses began to work with my physical strength, and told my body to stop shaking and start moving, and where to move, too!

Intuitively, I began to maneuver, step by step. I relaxed my feelings about the impending danger, and once I found the balance between my faith and my abilities, I got them to work together. One leading, the other following, and then exchanging roles, in order to get me down the rock safely. Slowly but surely I made it over the cliff, around the boulder, and finally down to the protected pathway that lead toward civilization.

The pain in my leg was a burning reminder of the jeopardy in which my life had been. If I had relied only on my mind, I probably would have panicked, screamed, and let go of the rope. If I had relied only on my physical strength, looking at the wounds on my legs, I should be shark bait, right now. I realized the throbbing in my leg was there to serve as a reminder of my free will, and God's promise.

As I inspected the wounds, I contemplated the lesson. I don't think faith, or physical ability, or knowledge could have worked by themselves, but when I was forced to bring all these worlds together, they worked in perfect unison, one to temper the other. What got me out of that situation was my mature faith; I was sure of it.

God was definitely getting my attention through pain, this time. I got what I asked for; more than just a metaphor. But you know me! I like to learn my lessons the hard way, and generally more than once. I realized that, without hope, what would be the point of expending any effort, anyway? Perhaps I could serve as hope to someone else. I got the day's message, and I was determined to use my pain for good somehow.

Once again standing on the civilized side of the cliffs, I was greeted by the applause of several sympathetic surfers who had been watching the events from below.

"Hey next time you wanna check out that cove, it's way easier to take a surf board, man. But that was some awesome determination. You've got some real cajones!" one shouted from the calmness of his floating board.

"Thanks," I smiled. "I appreciate you sharing that with me," I said, as I waved and limped down toward the sandy beach, leaving a red warning trail to all who might consider the climb that day.

This side of the cliff, the Winter's beach was giving way to a warm sunshine and the sandy shoreline was now spotted with beach towels, as well as curious onlookers.

As a young man was making his way up the sandy path with his five-year-old daughter in tow, he asked what had happened to me. Seeing as how I looked like I just came out of a battle, it was a little difficult for me to explain the beauty and peace of the lagoon with any credibility. The injuries on my legs and shoulders made it clear, without words, the other side of that pathway was no place for his daughter, right now. I explained to him, as another had explained to me, "The tides come up quick over there. If you can't time your retreat with the rising tides, don't go in, and be careful if you go it alone."

With that, I watched him turn his daughter around and point her back toward the safety of her beach towel. Something in me smiled, and

I realized it felt pretty good, after all, when my hurts were used to heal someone else, or keep someone from having to heal, altogether.

The lifeguard simply shook his head with that "What were you thinking?" kind of look, as I limped my way past his station.

♥The Ride Continues♥

I'd have given anything for a ride in God's big old limo, and almost as soon as I thought it, He was standing there with a clean towel for my leg, and a fresh bottle of cool Spring water for my salty mouth. I guess He figured I'd had enough lessons for the day. I made my way toward His car and I saw Him smiling.

"Looks like you've had a rough day," He said, with that familiar twinkle in His eyes. "Hop in, I wanna take you somewhere."

"Take me somewhere? Like this? I don't have—" and before the words came out of my mouth, there in the limo was a clean outfit, first-aid kit, and a laptop computer.

"Oh, the computer is so you can start typing your stories, like you promised. And the clothes; well, just run over to the showers and clean up a little. I'll wait for you," He said, getting into the driver's seat.

He was always there when I needed Him, but I could never predict when He was going to show up.

After cleaning up and bandaging my leg, I was ready for some lunch and a nice Starbuck's!

"No lunch, sorry," He shouted over his shoulder as we made our way down the street. "Now get to typing, like you promised Me, and I'll tell you when we get where were going. In the meantime, I'll see what I can do about your coffee," He said, as we speed off down the street.

After what seemed like hours, He suddenly stopped. Getting out of the car, He came around and opened my door.

"Here we are!"

Following his lead, I exited the car. Looking around, I could not tell exactly where we were.

"Now, do you need anything before I go?"

"Go? Go where? Where are You going and how am I supposed to know what I need. I thought that was Your job. And where do You think you're going? You can't leave me here in the middle of nowhere. I'm just starting to get the hang of this laptop computer deal and was just typing out a recipe for this whole Self♥Love thing," I said, standing there on what I perceived to be some random street corner.

"If you find that you do not have, it is because you do not ask Me for it," God said.

"Um, Okay," was my reply, as I stood shivering outside the car. I was tired, my leg still hurt, and the sun was beginning to set.

"Look, make it easy on yourself and just stay right around here until I get back. Use the things you've learned so far to find your way around while I'm gone. Have a little fun and don't wrinkle your forehead at me. Oh, and one more thing," He yelled out the window as He was pulling away. "While you're here, tell others about your road trip, so far. You'll help them feel better about their lives, and it will keep you out of trouble. Trust Me; it's called wisdom."

Then He handed me my laptop, and I watched Him speed off down the road. I stood there and squeezed my eyes shut. I just wanted to seek out His gentle face in my mind, and calm my shaking knees. It felt like I was back on that cliff again.

I tried my best to trust Him and just do what He told me to. I knew for certain now that He would help me get through whatever I didn't think I could get through on my own. I was sure He had done it earlier, when the waves were pounding at my back. So, even though I felt lost, and didn't know where to go or what to do, I was certain this couldn't be half as bad.

As soon as I pictured His face in my mind and heard His words, I felt this incredible peace come over me. It was sort of like that Spirit of power I felt, hanging on to that rope, over the rock cliff. Only this time it was filled with a sense of real love and self-discipline, and it took the place of timidity and fear within me. It made me feel so good about myself that I could open my eyes, and felt confident to start typing again.

Realizing I couldn't type standing up, I began to walk, without deliberate direction, while I thought about the stories I wanted to share. I found a bus stop bench and decided to sit there and, "Wait upon the Lord," as I was told to do.

Looking around, I noticed it was a kind of scary place to be all alone. But, pretty soon I was able to bypass the feelings of fear altogether, and focus all of me on sharing my gifts and talents in the stories I would write for other people's healing.

So, there I was. It was getting quite late in the evening and I was still sitting at this bus stop bench, freezing my tush off, with no money to even buy a hot Starbuck's, just waiting for God to come back. I closed my eyes and tried that eye-squeezing-shut thing again, hoping to create that feeling of peace and confidence I had gotten before. For once I was acting out of obedience and aligning myself with God's will for me on that day.

Sit still and wait upon the Lord, I heard over and over in my mind. I also heard *Lean not upon your own understanding, but upon Mine,* and when I opened my eyes, instead of getting that peaceful feeling, I noticed a girl sitting across the street from me.

It was pretty dark out, so it was hard to make out her face, but she kind of looked like...well, me. I noticed she was crying, and I was struggling with whether I should go over there and see if I could help, or do what God told me to do, and just sit still and wait for Him.

Actually, I remembered Him saying I was supposed to share what I had learned with other people, which is Self♥Love Potion ingredient number ten, sharing what you know.

 # Self♥Love Potion Ingredients

#1 ♥*Spirituality. Your personal connection to a higher power.*
#2 ♥*Knowing your Truths and accepting responsibility.*
#3 ♥*Letting go of envy.*
#4 ♥*Accepting the free will of others with Grace.*
#5 ♥*Listening.*
#6 ♥*Journaling.*
#7 ♥*Identifying Masks, revealing your true nature.*
#8 ♥*Symbols of Self♥Love.*
#9 ♥*Asking for Help!*
#10 ♥*Sharing what you know with others.*

So, there I was, trying to decide if I should go and help this girl or not. I was also thinking, *What if God comes back for me, doesn't see me sitting here, and thinks I'm all warm and cozy inside some coffee shop somewhere? He might take off and go run another errand and leave me out here freezing for hours.*

After weighing my options, I guess I ended up going with the "leaning not on my own understanding" part, rather than the "sitting still and waiting" part. So I walked across the street and sat down next to the girl. When I asked her if I could help, she just looked up at me, with these big ol' tears in her eyes, and said,

"Why does there have to be so much pain in this world?"

"Uh…well…oh, gosh, I'm probably not the right person you should be asking that question," I said, looking back at my park bench, reconsidering the whole helping idea.

As I watched her wipe the black mascara from her wet cheeks, I tried the eye-squeezing-shut thing again, hoping it would work. Suddenly my mouth opened up, and the words just began to flow.

"I guess we have pain mainly because of our gift of free will, and the free will choices of others in this world. See, we live in a world that is corrupted by sin and pain, so eventually we are bound to feel some of it in our lives," I said, offering her my coat. "But the good news is your pain is not always just about you, and you don't have to let your pain go to waste, or endure it alone, either!" I assured her, as I wrapped my coat around her.

I could feel the wind kicking up, and just out of reflex I looked over my shoulder to see if a large wave was going to accompany the gust. *That was really dumb,* I thought, standing there in the midnight air without my jacket. *Now I'm gonna freeze to death, and miss my ride, too.* But what was weird was that I was actually more comfortably warm without my jacket than I was before I offered it to the girl. *Great. Now I've got a fever,* I thought, looking down to check the bandages on my leg.

"You want some coffee?" the girl asked, as she pulled a stainless steel Starbuck's thermos from her purse. She must have seen the shocked look on my face, because she quickly added, "Oh, yeah, I work at Starbuck's on the weekends to earn some extra money."

She tried to steady her hand as she poured the coffee and said, "I've been working there to save up enough money to get my car fixed, but last night my boyfriend and I broke up, and, well, he took my heart and my car with him."

After handing me the cap full of coffee, she released another sob. I placed my arm around her heaving shoulders. I understood her pain completely. I began sharing my own stories of heartbreak and the healing that followed. After what seemed like hours, I finally saw the beginning of a smile forming on her saddened features. She realized she was not alone in her hurt and confusion about love.

Looking around, I suggested that the buses might have stopped running and watched that smile rapidly fade, once again, from her frail face. Now that we had spent so much time talking, it was too late, and too dangerous for her to walk home, safely, by herself. I felt kind of responsible, but more than a little helpless. What could I do? I didn't even know the area, or I would have at least offered to walk home with her. I had no money, so I couldn't call her a cab. All I could do was squeeze my eyes shut in faith and hope it worked again.

As soon as I opened my eyes, I saw them—the unmistakable headlights of that big black limo!

"Thank God," I heard myself say, and had to smile at the truth of the words.

"Hey look, that's my ride coming up the street," I know there's going to be room for at least one more person in there."

I knew God was returning for me, but sometimes He came back with an entire limo full of other people, too. But in that moment, I found it easy to offer her my ride. I was willing to sit on that bus bench as long as it took for God to care of my new friend. He would come back for me. I knew he would because He always did.

"Look, it may be a little cramped in there, but why don't you let God give you a lift home tonight? At least it's safer than going on alone. I'll be perfectly alright sitting right here until He comes back for me" I said, signaling the limo. "I know it may not change everything in your life all at once, but you can ask God for His business card and maybe you guys can work out a transportation deal until you can get your car back. He would be more than willing to give you a lift and help you work things out." I said, continuing to flag down the limo.

Looking at me in protest she said, "No, I couldn't take your ride and leave you sitting here. I would feel horrible about that. And besides, how do you know He would come back for you, anyway?"

"Trust me," I said, and as soon as those words came out of my mouth, I realized, I was beginning to sound just like Him! As soon as God pulled up to the curb, I explained the story to Him. With a radiant smile, He said,

"I am so proud of your progress. See, you don't always have to learn through pain when you are paying attention to the assignments. Now, hop on in. There's plenty of room for the both of you."

It was as if He had anticipated my guest's arrival. He had the car cleaned and freshened and, as we both hopped in the back seat, the girl and I exchanged phone numbers, and we are still in touch to this day.

Over the years God made some incredible changes in her life and I get all the praises for introducing the two of them! I just love how that works. Funny thing though, she said God never picked her up in that limo again. She tells me He always picks her up on a Harley. Go figure!

It didn't take long for me to discover that when God dropped me off on some random street corner, He never really left me alone, either. During those cold night hours, or anytime He left me to my own devices, those were the times He was planning something extraordinarily special for someone in my life or for me. He was just going on up ahead to make sure all the preparations were being taken care of just so—such a perfectionist.

Many times those people I chose to help out while I was waiting for God to return had actually been dropped off there on purpose for me, by God, to kind of help me help myself while He was away! I'm learning to enjoy His sense of humor.

He always returned, just like He said He would, and I learned to trust Him in this way. I really enjoyed it when He would return with company. I think God was probably multi-tasking during those times—I mean, since we're all going in the same direction, anyway. Kind of like us right now.

As you read the pages in this book, you are taking this journey with me. What your destination is I can't say for sure. But I do know that you are searching for something more than what you are right now.

> ♥Everyone's Self♥Love Potion comes from an inspiration to be more than they think they can be on their own. ♥

There is definitely something more out there, and sometimes we just need a moment to figure it out and a little lift along the way to finding it.

God is unquestionably the driving force behind my life's ride. Trust me! You'll end up in a better place than you are right now if you will just do what I did. Sit there for a while and paint your toenails (guys, you can just polish your shoes or something) and trust that God has heard your prayers, and He will answer them when He is good and ready. All we have to do is show up, shut up, and listen.

Chapter Seven

Chapter Seven

♥ The Most Volatile Ingredient? ♥
♥ Self ♥ Love Potion Ingredient #11
♥ The Ultimate Romantic Formula
♥ Girls Guys and Gossip

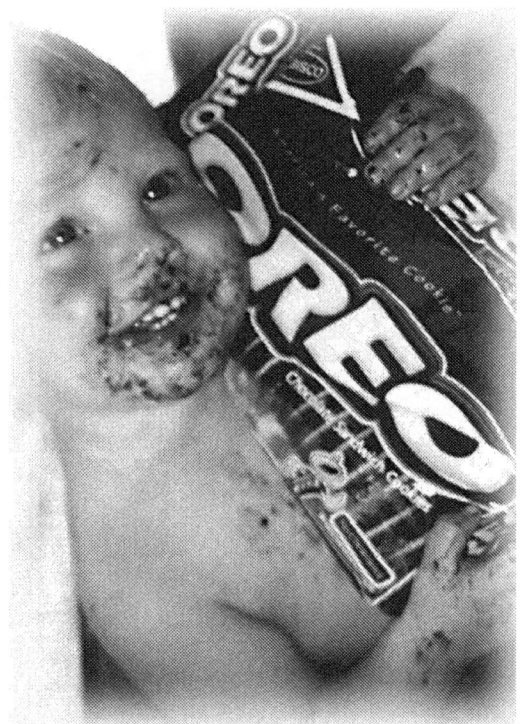

♥ Romantic love; is it anything more than just the perception of
the romantic? ~

The Most Volatile Ingredient?

My girlfriend asked me why I used the word volatile instead of unpredictable or unstable, impulsive or even erratic when I was talking about Self♥Love Potion ingredient number eleven, which is the blending of Self♥Love with romantic love.

 # Self♥Love Potion Ingredients

#1 ♥ *Spirituality. Your personal connection to a higher power.*
#2 ♥ *Knowing your Truths and accepting responsibility.*
#3 ♥ *Letting go of envy.*
#4 ♥ *Accepting the free will of others with Grace.*
#5 ♥ *Listening.*
#6 ♥ *Journaling.*
#7 ♥ *Identifying Masks, revealing your true nature.*
#8 ♥ *Symbols of Self♥Love.*
#9 ♥ *Asking for Help!*
#10 ♥ *Sharing what you know with others.*
#11 ♥ *Blending of Self♥Love with romantic love.*

My response to that question is that the term volatile best describes what "romantic" love can do to a weak Self♥Love Potion if it is added in "incompatible" proportions to the recipe. Personally, I like to add two parts God's love to one part Romantic Love. I was also quick to remind my girlfriend that volatile and violent are two different words.

When I was following my own romantic agenda of finding a hero to save me from the responsibility of being me, I continued to have dire results with those romantic ingredients that just could not sweeten my potions (or fulfill the conditions) to my satisfaction. I was so sure that romantic love was the final and most important ingredient in my Self♥Love Potion that no matter how much I hurt, I just kept adding, mixing, and tasting.

It wasn't until I realized that it was the "pursuit" of romantic love that was so unforgiving to my recipes, and not the love itself. The pursuit is what had made me a slave. A slave to the search. The only person Falling apart was me, because in my efforts to control everyone else's actions and fix their problems, I created enormous problems for myself. My sacred kitchen, the place where I was supposed to be creating Self♥Loving recipes, well, it was a disaster area. Instead of a hard hat, you needed a hardened heart to enter my laboratory.

Sometimes it is hard not to feel trapped by our circumstances, and I realized the search and momentary attainment of romance was only a temporary escape from a broken heart's reality. Those moments of being swept off my feet felt so good that I actually became drunk with that temporary perception of love.

Have you ever tried to bake a cake while you were intoxicated? Try making a Self♥Love recipe under the influence of chemistry and romance. Even with the directions staring me right in the face, I still added too much of this and not enough of that and absolutely none of some of the most important ingredients.

The recipes always looked like they were going to turn out fabulous, but as long as I was under the drunkenness of a fleeting romantic influence, the final result was always disastrous!

True romance feels really good, but let me be clear on one thing…Romance is NOT REQUIRED to make a Self♥Love Potion work. If you're not standing on your own two feet when romance does come along, then you're going to end up settling for something inside of your relationship to make room for the expectation. Romance can have such an intoxicating effect on our chemistry, that we may find ourselves addicted to its immediate effect so much so that we fail to consider the long-term side effects on our relationships, as we continue to crave more and more of that romantic stimulus from our partner (who, by the way, will never be able to satiate that need for you).

Romance, in and of itself, is such an unstable ingredient that I don't even add it to my Self♥Love Potions anymore. I have separate jars marked "Romance only" and I keep them a good distance from any of my other Self♥Love recipes so as not to mix them by mistake.

Romance can change the flavor of a good Self♥Love Potion to rancid in a heartbeat or make it even sweeter than the syrup you originally had in mind. Therefore, I consume romance as a side dish to my Self♥Love recipes, and when I do, it tastes more like the true blessing it was intended to be.

True romance can be a real gift from God's little angels. It is good to have an idea of what you are looking for, romantically, but keep your ingredients in the proper order. Romance should be somewhat down the list if you are already struggling with a healthy Self♥Loving recipe. Sure, a good dose of romance can certainly inspire you and even help you heal from time to time, but romance is no substitute for an honest to goodness "Self♥Love recipe," as self-love saves and revives!

♥The Ultimate Romantic Formula

So what about the fairytale itself? Well, with that little disclaimer being made, let us talk a little about the gaiety and true enchantment of pure, unadulterated, good ole-fashion romance!

I suppose if I could pick the perfect time of year to indulge in an ultimate romantic formula (for me anyway), I should like its magic to originate from the resting months of Winter, when my wisdom and introspection are at their highest peak.

I guess I would start experimenting with my recipe around February because it's the dead center of Winter and a highly reflective time of the heart.

Let's see, it would be raining outside and the wind would be howling. I would probably order the vegetable soup and he would have the chicken noodle with half a sandwich.

When he smiled at me, it would seem somehow familiar, as if I could see God reflected in his very presence. Our conversation would flow effortlessly, with several hours passing before either one of us even glanced at our watch. His eyes, crystal blue, of course, would mirror the reflection of his light blue flannel shirt. He'd have a look of strength about him and I would contemplate the ability of his arms. Would they be strong enough to hold me up, protect me, and yet gentle enough to touch me with tender care?

He would be honest and forthright in his questioning, making certain not to ask too much, while learning all he could. His edge would be somewhat softened by his calm presence. As he smiled, he would reach out to take his napkin, softly brushing my hand while stating more than asking if I…

"Trust that God's unconditional love was sufficient for a peaceful, purposeful life while here on earth?"

At this point I would take a moment, a deep breath, and then reply, "Yes, I trust God's love is sufficient for me, if it is all God desires for my life." Then I would lean in and whisper in my classic style, "But I still have romantic delusions of earthly love nevertheless!"

He would smile, then motion for that romantically delusional part of me to continue as he'd ask, "In the form of a living, breathing man, I imagine?"

"Yes, that's kind of what I had in mind"

"What would he be like? This romantic man you dream of? Some traits, qualities…" he'd ask.

"Oh, that's easy. He would be a great wordsmith, and as he expressed his Spiritual relationship and commitments to God by sharing his life with me, his eyes would misrepresent nothing. I'd see the world as God intended me to see it with him. His heart would do me a great service by allowing God's unconditional love to flow through him and to me. Of course I'd like him to be financially stable and move with self-confidence and determination through life…"

♥ Can Fairytales Come True?

Just by a chance assignation, I found myself in the middle of Winter, under the exact circumstances described above. There I was, sitting across the table from a man with whom I had **no** expectations, simply enjoying the ♥moments of Winter's wisdom whispered from his lips that day.

There have been others that have tried to discuss God's lessons of love on a deep and meaningful level, but today would be the day that I would actually understand the reciprocated words. Perhaps because of the introspection of Winter's wisdom (timing), or perhaps it was because I had spent the past several Winters learning my lessons and was now able to feel the intensity of a Loving Voice.

As we talked and I listened I realized that my understanding of what it would be like to be romantically loved by a God fearing man was as tenuous as puffing on a dandelion. His words struck to my very core. I realized that romance and reality are one in the same thing for a man who respects the Lord.

"I believe that whatever a man wants, he must give it first," he said. "That's how I believe a man should love, but he can only do this for a woman who has chosen to love herself first," he added.

"Ahhh, a woman familiar with her own Self♥Love Potion recipe," I said, smiling and nodding.

We had both shared similar lessons in love's travels; romantically loving out of need and fear, rather than unconditional peace and faith. We both laughed at the understanding of our similar broken pieces and how we chose to let God heal them. We both believed that if either of us ever wanted to really taste the piquancy of unconditional love and truth, we had to start with giving these things to ourselves first and look to God for the right recipes.

As he continued to share his view of the man as typically being the head of the household protector, I felt my head nodding in agreement.

"I believe he is commissioned to fight for more than just the household," he continued. "He needs to protect, not just with his body size and physical strength, but with his mind, his faith and his heart. If he is to have love, he must serve love and protect love with his whole being, don't you think?"

I was appreciating this conversation as much as a child might appreciate a scavenger hunt, and I asked him to continue, as I captured every word with my imagination! He smiled that delightful smile and obliged.

"Well, if you're asking me personally, I would put my woman above myself, never allowing any circumstance to occur that would diminish my desire to know and love her better each day. I believe we are all created in our Lord's image, but in her, I would see all my favorite things of my Lord, all the wonder of life, the beauty, and power of Love, and the evidence of things hoped for, felt maybe, but not yet seen.

Since I know God surely loves me, and I believe love is reciprocal, my desire is to return God's Love for me by loving the woman of my life, just as my Lord said, 'Love your mate as Christ Loves the Church.'

So, is that to say that I would lay down my life for her? Well, I guess that means I would. But you know, even that would not tell her the depth or width of how I feel my Lord loves me. When I really think about it, I would say that I would give my woman the very heart out of my chest, but unless there came a time that would be what is asked of me, my heart would stay right beside her, and beat for her.

Yeah, our love would be a testimony to the love that I feel from God, and a witness to others of what God has for them. I don't know. For whatever reason, even though I've waited this long, I still believe that love is not only possible, but love is real, and I believe it does exist!"

"Wow," was all my eyes could speak. This guy has to be drunk on his own romantic potion, I thought. There is no way in the world a woman could make a man feel like that. He has to already have that love inside of him. Certainly, it would have to be "Spirit" inspired, I thought.

My delayed reaction must have gone undetected because he continued to bite on his sandwich, intermittently, while he thought, then continued to speak using metaphors and symbols one minute, and knowledge and skill the next. He was being precise and direct, and it was stunning to both watch and hear.

Since each side of the brain has its own language (and he was definitely combining both), I had to take a moment to absorb all that he was saying without choking on my soup. This man I was sitting across from was mesmerizing. He communicated his thoughts as if he was solving a problem. (As a rule, I think men generally deal with feelings by logic, and their ordinary language usually seems, well...sterile and unimaginative, or kind of objective to me.) But this guy was not trying to guide me to a correct solution; he was just communicating his truths in a smooth subjective language of intimacy that I found both enlightening and rewarding, as I drank him in.

"So you're as romantically delusional as I am," I said, playing with my soup. "So, tell me more about what this woman, the one you would love like that. What is she going to have to do to attract your attention? I mean, since no one has managed to attract your heart so far? You sure she even exists?" I said, half-joking, but eager to hear his reflection.

"Well, I trust there will only be one woman for me, and I will continue to wait upon the Lord to plant that seed of love within me for her. Love is a gift, and I have to choose it. My soul mate, the one with whom I ask God to make me "one flesh," not just with physical oneness, but also Spiritual, emotional, and intellectual oneness. I want to be intimate with her on every level of her being. Anyway, when she does arrive, I'm not sure I know exactly what she will look like. I guess men are drawn to a woman with their eyes first, so I suppose she will be attractive to discover. That's how I ended up in your Bible study group you know," he added, with a pause and broad smile for emphasis.

"I hope you don't take that the wrong way. I was just having fun with the idea of your visual beauty when I joined your group. I think you're a great small group leader," he continued, letting go of the fear that he had crossed a friendship boundary.

Flashing him a wide approving grin, "Okay, so she'll be like fireworks; smoke and thunder then, right?" I teased laughingly, prodding him to continue.

"Let's see," he said, raising his napkin to the corner of his smile, while nodding his approval. "I guess she would probably be visually attractive, fit, and physically desirable," adding a wink, just to watch me squirm. "But first we would be Spiritually compatible, and have similar life purposes, as well. She'd have a quick wit, for sure; probably clever, wise, maybe a little sophisticated. I bet she would be able to transition easily from gaiety to somber and sensual, and back again. I believe she would be the kind of woman who had above average Spiritual standards, to which she held herself accountable."

My silence must have signaled him to continue on with his list, but actually I was still thinking about what he had said about how he ended up in my Bible study group.

"Okay…well, I guess I could go down the list of confident, reverent, humble, optimistic, accomplished, blah, blah, blah…But one thing's for sure…when I stare into the eyes and heart of her wonderful soul, and start to kiss her, I'll never want to stop!" he said, taking in a deep breath and another bite of his sandwich.

"Good God! That has certainly got to be some girl! You've been wait-ing how many years for her?" I said, giggling, and slurping my vegetable soup.

"That statement is a credit to your lack of patience, my dear Cynthia," he said, his voice cutting through all my defenses. "I believe love is a gift from God. Once given and accepted, it is as permanent and as strong as death...so I am willing to wait as long as it takes for the right one, if that's God will for my life. Do you know what I mean? I want the kind of love that cannot be purchased or earned, but just as our salvation in Jesus is a gift that is first going to be given to me, then, if I choose it, I will be able to share it with the woman of my dreams. I'll tell you one thing; she will definitely know her Lord loved her, and that my Lord and Savior has given her a gift!" he proclaimed, taking another bite of his sandwich and pointing his finger into his chest.

"You? What makes you any different than every other man out there?" I said mockingly. "That's a kind of egotistical perspective, don't you think?

Laughing out loud and puffing up his chest, he said "Yeah, I guess I did get a little carried away, but I mean, heck, wouldn't you want to be loved like that? If God gave some guy the ability to love you like that, wouldn't you consider him a gift?

"Well, I..." was all that came out of my mouth.

"I think I would be a gift to her because I have chosen to give my life to the Lord, and two years ago I offered my life as a vehicle through which the Lord may love one of his precious daughters. I guess I'll be showing God how much I love HIM by loving his most precious cre-ation, and if I am going to allow myself to be used by God like that, He is going to send me His very best. Hopefully, she will consider me her gift as much as I will consider her mine!"

Clearing my throat, I offered, "Well, I guess it's possible for you to have ALL the desires of your heart met, but my experience tells me—" but before I could finish, he interjected, with warmth,

"When I let the Lord love a woman like that through me, she's going to know that promises can be kept...that love is real...and that she is worthy of that kind of love." Then he looked me dead in the eyes, leaned in, and smiled.

Averting my eyes and folding the napkin nervously in my lap, I tilted my head questioningly and, returning his stare,

"So, let's say you do meet this woman of your dreams and she turns out to be less than what you expected; what then?"

As he sat back in his chair and finished wiping the corner of his mouth, he replied, "I'm not going to worry too much about what I want; I am just going to focus on what God wants for her, after I've made the choice to love her. I trust my needs will be met by doing so. My biggest dilemma is in choosing to act on the gift of love once it's placed inside of me. It goes back to that romantic delusion you were talking about. No man likes rejection," he murmured, under yet another bite of sandwich. "Remember Solomon?" he asked, as he took a large gulp of his iced tea.

"Of course I know of Solomon; the most romantic figure in the Bible! My Gosh; but you know who I found just as fascinating? The Queen of Sheba. Did you know that she was the first woman with a past to be spoken about in the Bible," I said, returning to my meal. "She brought the richest and wisest man in the world to his knees with her love."

"Yes, that's true," he continued. "However, the Queen of Sheba had such a confidence about her, according the stories I've read, anyway, that her sex appeal was not her strength; it was a gentle fusion of her strengths and vulnerability—her Self♥Love, more than anything else, I think. She was a woman who knew her own self worth," he said, matter-of-factly.

"But you got me off-track, I was talking about Solomon," he said, lifting his eyebrow to recall the romantic figure he was about to quote. "Now, Solomon; God really spoke of romantic and real love through

Solomon: 'Seal me in your heart with permanent betrothal, for Love is as strong as death!' Just fascinating! See, I hope I can love like that. Here this man had everything in the world, yet I believe the Lord was showing Solomon the power of romance, as well as the sacrifices that go along with it. Once I accept the choice to be committed, I already know I will desire her with every fiber in my being. She is going to get my attention, however God chooses for her to do it, be it looks, talent, or Spirit. But once we commit to each other, I will adore her, cherish her, need her, admire her, and be blessed with her, no matter what she looks like, or how many of my delusions are shattered by the reality of her."

He paused for a moment noticing the expression on my face, and then continued, "Hey, I'm just saying I 'want' to love like this. At least I'm willing to give it my best shot, but I know I can't do it alone. It's going to take the strength of God to help me through the rough times, and I am sure there will be rough times; but that's just the reality of life."

A slight tearing in my eye and quivering to my lips announced my truth. I had no idea what it would be like to be loved like that. I suppose that's when the protective part of my heart kicked in and whispered, "Hey, he's 41 and still single. Maybe it's perfectly safe for him to live in his own romantic fantasy of waiting for a woman who doesn't exist, so he can justify being intimately unavailable."

Hmmmm, I thought as I reconciled my lack of knowledge and avoided the flood of tears welling up inside of me. "I guess it must scare the heck out of you to actually get close to a woman then, huh?" I said, wiping the tear before he could notice the wetness on my cheek. *"I suppose if you ever did choose and it didn't work out, then you'd be ruined."*

"No," he said, matter-of-factly, looking me dead in the eyes. "But it might be scary for someone like you, who I know has chosen love and has been deeply hurt by love's promise."

Then there was silence. I didn't know whether to excuse myself from the table, or just continue to pretend I wasn't paying attention to his deep stare. I felt as if he were looking right into the heart of me.

"These are not just mere words that I'm spilling out on you—they are coming from my heart, my soul and my Spirit. I'm telling you, I will know love as a fact, and as a promise, to and from our God. I think you believe the same thing. Don't give up that dream, Cynthia. Love is real. You just have to be ready to RECEIVE love the next time it comes around to you. Just because I make the choice to give my love, that doesn't guarantee me that it will be received. It's scary for me, too."

Shuddering at the thought that he could see that deeply into my heart, I tried an adaptive approach to our communication. "So, you think God will just plop this gift of love in your lap one day? Just like that—out of nowhere?"

"Something like that," he nodded. "I've felt the potential before, but, for whatever reasons—my own fears, issues, or broken pieces—I didn't choose the gift. I came really close, once, but she wasn't capable of receiving it. By the time I figured it out I had already learned some painful lessons. I've just kept moving forward, learning and growing closer to God, and trusting that the next time the choice is given I'll have the courage to act on it—and she will have the courage to accept it! I take the commitment of love pretty seriously, you know," he continued, almost weakly.

"This life that we are given is a gift, but it is also a test, to see what we will do with it," he said, lifting my chin in his hand. "True love isn't passive; it demands a response. It grows in character, and in satisfying ways. Your heart is not broken as much as you think it is, Cynthia. As a matter of fact," he said, his fingertips lifting my chin just a bit higher, so he could see directly into my eyes, "I believe your heart is one that came directly from God's."

Squishing my brows together and freeing myself from his reach, I wrinkled my forehead and countered softy, "O…K…R i i g h t!"

"No, I'm serious. I think before He decided to let you go out to play in the rest of His creation, He must have thought, 'One final touch to set this woman apart as my own; I will make her heart out of a piece of my very own.' Yes, I'm sure that's what He must have been thinking. What I see in you when I watch you teach your classes is God showing off all His best. You are a reflection of all the love that my Lord has for His children." His eyes glimmered as I allowed him to gaze at me.

Then, I smiled, and there was laughter. I blushed and replied, "Thank you; that was really sweet thing to say."

He silently watched me for a moment. Then a light of acknowledgment flashed across his face. "I'm extremely impressed with your courage, Cynthia," he said tapping his fingers on the wooden tabletop.

"What words could I possibly use to communicate to you just how beautiful I think your heart is, to those of us that watch you? Yes, even those broken pieces you try to hide, so well. Should I compare your heart to the ocean, which I know you love a great deal, or how about the forests, the stars…moonlight? I could compare the compassion of it to great, noble causes and sacrifices with ease, but what do I have to compare the beauty of the courage of your heart?"

After a few moments of raised eyebrows, he snapped his fingers. "I don't really have the words. Not because of a lack of effort; it's just because they simply don't exist! That's it! There ARE no words. So, I'll just leave it at that," he said, satisfied with his answer.

"God didn't put you here alone, and don't you ever give up on the hope that He made another just for you," he said enthusiastically. "It's going to take courage to choose love again, but that is the most beautiful part of you; your faith! Yup, that's it, that's your courage; your faith!" he said, smacking his lips in contentment.

I laughed to myself in complete understanding of the words he had chosen not to use. He placed his hands flat on the table, signaling it was time to go.

Immediately, I assessed the change in body language, looked at my watch, and offered him a way out. "Oh, gosh, it's time to go. I can't believe we spent so much time."

"Oh, yes…please, don't let me keep you. I've got an appointment to get to, myself," he said, grinning a slightly silly grin. Reaching for the check he said,

"I treasure this walk with you, Cynthia. You encourage me, and I do appreciate the moments you take for our friendship"

Both hearts anticipating the finish, we asked ourselves, as we excited the restaurant, *Could this be love in motion?*

Eureka! Sweet romance, dipped in committed, Spiritual fire! Renewed faith in idealistic, impractical, passionate, romantic love! What a fine sugary syrup of a potion! The thing I had given up the pursuit of had now found its way, full circle, to me, once I had stopped looking for it!

> ♥ In retrospect, I believe that it wasn't until I got to the place where I was able to surrender the pursuit of romantic love to God's perfect love, that I was given a very special taste of God's unconditional love. ♥

The learning of what God calls "unconditional love" required me to add forgiveness and Grace to some of the older recipes I had been developing. I've ended up producing some of the most essential Self♥Love recipes of all times from those lessons.

As I began sharing those potions and recipes with others, I found those bottles marked Grace, Compassion, and Forgiveness, would never empty, no matter how much of them I gave away. I marked those bottomless bottles with big red hearts, to remind me that they are full, and perfect, and contain very special ingredients!

All I had to do with those recipes was to share them with others, and they would remain full, forever.

♥It is so amazing to me that such simple acts of compassion for others could produce such profound effects in my own life. ♥

~Girls, Guys & Gossip ~

My Girlfriend~ Elegant Spirit in an Original Form

This graceful creature moves through life, tossing her raven black hair, filling the air with laughter, and flashing warmth from across a crowded room with her large, doe-shaped eyes.

Her hospitable nature is unmistakable. Her frailty is disguised in razor-sharp attentive ways; yet, always, she is at ease.

In the slightest moments with her, this soft, lovable creature with milky white skin will expose your truth.

In her persistence, you're made aware that she does not exist in ordinary time. Her reality is that of Spiritual freedom.

She is the very breath of God, in her domestic nature, and she stands firm and protective on this ground.

There is no escape from a focused message, delivered by a dimpled smile, a raised brow, and a hand strategically placed on her left hip.

Her fire refuses anything but truth, and God help the receiver of her graceful pointed finger.

It pleasures her to sample indulgences of this world, alluring as any bright light to a moth. Yet, her peace of mind comes from a heart that beats for only one.

For his gifts, she offers him a resolute and devoted embrace. Only she understands the depth of him, and he gladly showers her with artful pleasures, as she lifts him up in honor.

She is my friend, an elegant Spirit in an original form. God was clear in His design of her, and for this and more, I praise Him.

~C

♥ The Girls ♥

Several months after that lunch meeting, I found myself discussing my encounter with my girlfriends. There in my living room, I sat with my two best friends, trying to explain the reflections of love I was getting from my first encounter, and every encounter I've had since, with this man I now refer to as *"A Loving Voice."*

"I met him several months ago in my Bible study group," I said, responding to their inquiry as to where this man who was capturing my interest and my heart had first appeared. "…Honest, I didn't even think about dating him when we first met. Remember back when I decided to stop dating all together? Well, a few months later is when I met him," I said, cheerfully

"Oh, yeah, isn't that when you got involved in some sort of ministry at church, too?" one girlfriend asked.

"That's what I'm trying to tell you. That's how it happened!" I said, smiling at their stares of anticipation. "I showed up at church on a Wednesday night, because someone at the church called me and asked me if I would be willing to lead a small fellowship group in my home. When I got to church, we were told to gather around certain tables. One thing lead to another and, next thing you know, I've got ten people meeting in my living room every Wednesday evening, sharing and learning about God's loving recipes and His outline for choosing a mate"

"So, how **do** you choose the right mate?" my worldly girlfriend interjected.

"Well, according to this study, God said that it's not good for us to be alone, whether we marry or not. So, if you're a Christian, you should choose AFTER you decide to make Christ the center of your life. After that, having a relationship is the next most important decision a person can make," I said, realizing I may have offered more information, from a personal perspective, than my girlfriend was asking for.

"Whatever. I see people get married to the wrong people all the time. I don't think it matters if they're Christians or not," she countered.

"Yeah, I can see your point, and a lot of people do get married to the wrong people, or get married at the wrong time. And, in this study, I recognized that the courting and engagement part of the relationship is a very important part of the process, and being with someone who shares your beliefs is a great way to lessen the possibility of marrying the wrong person—in my case, AGAIN! That's why I wanted to take the class in the first place. I want to be married again, but not just for the sake of being married; I want to be with the right partner for the rest of my life," I added.

"I think men tend to fear the whole courting process, in general," my Christian girlfriend offered, "especially here in California."

"Yeah, they pass right over the courting to get to the honey of a relationship, so I just save myself the trouble of fighting with 'em and give it to 'em right up front, if you know what I mean," my worldly girlfriend added, snapping her fingers and causing us both to roll our eyes.

"I don't know. I think courting and even an engagement can look like an all or nothing proposition for most men. I think that concept is what scares the heck out of them, especially if they don't know what they want," I said.

"I think you should know by the second date whether or not a guy is marriage material or not," my Christian girlfriend added.

"Wait a minute, Sista, I never said nothin' 'bout no marriage... 'mate'...capital M-A-T-E is what I am talking bout," my worldly girl-friend exclaimed, waving a pointed finger.

"Oh, 'Whatever' to both you guys," I said, as I removed a box of pop-corn from the kitchen cabinet.

"I'm talking about a life partner; a deep and meaningful kind of rela-tionship. The kind that's fulfilling for both sides of the relationship. And I have to agree that, if you're following God's principles, it can save a lot of time for a woman, who can waste literally months on the wrong man, and it saves time and money for a man, who can waste energy and income courting the wrong woman!"

"According to Marian Williamson, we are lovable and whole and desirable from the day that breath of life came to our bodies, and our perception only becomes altered when we look for love in another per-son," my worldly girlfriend replied, pausing for a moment to see if I would respond. Then she continued, as I placed one of the bags of pop-corn into the microwave. "So, are you telling me God's gonna choose your partner for you?"

"No that's not what I'm learning. And I really don't think it works that way, but I think God gives us guidance, principles, and direction for choosing a partner that makes the process a whole lot easier than what I was doing before. I am not looking for myself in another person, and following God's principles allows us to learn what real love is. Sometimes that means learning to love ourselves in a different way, first," I said.

"Yeah, okay, whatever...anyway, so back to your story about how you and this guy that's been making you all goofy-eyed met. He probably had wings, huh?" my worldly girlfriend teased, as I continued to check on the popcorn.

"No, not exactly. First of all, I wasn't looking at any of the men in my Bible study group as a potential boyfriend, anyway. I was just participat-ing in the group because, I felt called to be there. But I do remember meeting him the first time. I got this peaceful feeling right away from him…"

"Okay, okay, so what happened next," she said, letting out a sigh and waving her hand back and forth, as if she were becoming impatient with me.

"Okay, well, so here we were, becoming friends and learning about the Bible together, and one day we were having lunch, talking about the subject of love, from God's perspective as opposed to the world's view, and all of a sudden I just started tearing up. It was so cool, 'cause he wasn't saying these things for my benefit, he was just sharing one of his own Self♥Loving recipes honestly and openly with me," I continued, as I placed a bowl on the table between us.

"Well, so, what happened?" my worldly girlfriend urged, as she filled the bowl with hot, buttery, popped kernels and, scooping up a handful, happily flung them into her mouth.

"Well, later that night, I started thinking about our lunch meeting and what it would be like to be loved the way he was describing it…you know what I mean? Then, all of a sudden, I just started balling my eyes out thinking…God…"

"Oh my gosh, this is so romantic, it's like that movie, When Harry Met Sally," she said, reaching for more popcorn. "So, what happened next?"

"Ummmm, well, anyway…that's when I kind of thought this guy's got a great Spirit, and it was very attractive to me."

"So, you fell in love right then," my worldly girlfriend chirped, trying to contain her emotions, while catching the popcorn as she flipped them into her mouth.

My Christian girlfriend (reaching over and lightly but purposefully whacking my worldly girlfriend on the shoulder) said, "Would you just be quiet for a minute and let her finish, for heaven's sake? If you keep interrupting, she is never going to get the story out!"

Then, as she turned her face back toward mine, they both leaned forward and asked, "So…is that when you fell in love?"

"No, silly. Well, yes and no. I don't know…I think so. I kind of fell in love with his Spiritual maturity I guess more than anything else. I had never met a man so full of God's Spirit. I wasn't actually romantically connected to him in any way, but he just had such a beautiful calming presence that something inside of me just really craved his company. Besides, I wasn't really looking for romance at that time. I was just getting the hang of being happy with me, you know? But, yeah, there was definitely something going on between us."

"Okay, okay, so what happened next? Get to the good stuff," my worldly girlfriend urged, as she continuing to flip the kernels through the air.

"Okay! Wait! I'm getting there. Geez! But, let me tell you what happened first. One evening after our Bible study class, he stayed over to help with the dishes, and next thing you know we found ourselves sitting right here on this couch, just enjoying each other's company, and we starting to talk about more personal stuff, 'til late into the night. It was really nice to just be friends with a guy instead of the whole fifty questions in three dates kind of thing, ya know? Anyway, next thing you know, my knight in shining armor casting came crashing down off the wall! I pulled the big screen TV away from the wall and there was plaster everywhere. I told him I had had that casting for years, and it looked like my knight in shining armor just crashed and burned!"

Squishing the puffy corn between their fingers, my girlfriends listened, intently, as I continued.

"So then, he gets up from the couch, he takes my hand in his, and looks me dead in the eye and says, 'No. Perhaps your knight has simply served his purpose, and maybe, quite possibly it is my turn?"

"Oh, my gosh. I just got chills!" my worldly girlfriend whispered, as she reached for my hand. My Christian girlfriend joined her with a, "Praise the Lord."

"I know, I know, I got chills too when it happened. It was just so weird. We both could kind of feel something happening between us, but we didn't want to rush into some romantic fantasy that each of us was creating. We needed time to think and pray about what we felt happening. We both knew we had some real lifestyle differences that could create a future roadblock towards a marriage-bound relationship. And we both knew we were interested in a life mate, and not just a casual dating lifestyle, so we were taking the time to be discerning, and paying attention to the red flags. I mean, that's why we were in that bible study group in the first place: to learn discernment in relationships. Anyway, right after he had held my hand in his, he went home."

"What?!? He didn't kiss you? Weren't you just dying to kiss him? Oh my gosh, I can't believe you let him leave. I would have just ripped his clothes off and done him right there and then," my worldly friend said, with a heavy breath.

"Would you get your mind out of the gutter for one second and let her finish the story already!" my Christian friend commanded. "Go on, honey, I'm listening. So, what happened next?"

"Well," I continued, "after we played with the idea of the possibility of building a relationship between us and took the time to consider whether or not we wanted to risk our growing friendship, he asked me out on a genuine date and I accepted."

"Well I hope he at least took you some place romantic and expensive, after going home acting all chivalrous or whatever," my worldly girl-friend said, under her breath, as she judgmentally clicked her fingernails back and forth on the popcorn bowl. "Leaving you standing there in your own doorway all goo-goo-eyed and what not."

"You don't give anyone a break do you?" I responded, as I grabbed the bowl from her clutches. "We were both kind of on guard. We kept it very simple, at first. He asked me to church, and then a walk on the beach, and then brunch, and so on. The opportunity between us was becoming very clear but there were still some lifestyle issues that had to be addressed."

"Didn't you say you went to Catalina or something, to really be alone, and really pray about entering into a relationship with this guy?" my Christian girlfriend asked, more for our worldly girlfriend's benefit than for my response.

"Yeah, as a matter of fact, I did. I wanted to let God lead me, but I had to listen for His direction, so, I took off for a couple of days to really pray about it. Sitting atop that mountain, I really felt at peace with my ability to make good decisions. It was an awesome feeling to let God lead me. I mean, not that I was expecting God to make this the perfect relationship, but I was expecting God to lead me through it, no matter how it turned out. I felt really joyful for the opportunity."

"Yeah, you were probably hyperventilating from the climb," my worldly friend whispered.

"No, seriously; I did feel great and those dolphins, ohhhhhh; I just sat there for what must have been hours and prayed for discernment. Not just about having a boyfriend, but for every direction of my life,"

"Well what did the good lord have to say to you while you were sitting up there on that hill? Did he like, light a bush on fire or something and tell you to date this guy?" my worldly friend teased, but only half joking.

"No, there were no burning bushes, but I did get this feeling like God was telling me He sent this guy to me for a very important reason, but that only time and the voice in my heart was going to tell if it's love, or simply an added life's lesson toward 'faith in real love' once again.' I said, smiling.

"So at least you knew that you weren't just rushing head first into another relationship, huh?" my Christian girlfriend asked. "Now, how did he feel about you? The same way?" She continued with a tone in her voice that implied a real interest in hearing the answer.

"Ummm, well, he did tell me that I had never left him, from our first lunch together. But just because love is sent, that does not mean it has to be received. I think love is all about making a choice, and then making a commitment to that choice." I said, as I placed my hand over my heart.

"Wow, how romantic…So, when did you guys decide to go for it, you know, the love part?" my worldly friend urged, with a twinkle in her eye that begged for more information.

"Well, we talked about how we felt about each other. Since we were sharing a passion for the same God on the same level, it felt really kind of safe and really good to spend quality time together. Our goal was to just focus on following the Spirit down a path that may have ended up being a blessing for both our hearts, no matter where we ended up romantically. Who knows for sure what's going to happen? But I'll tell you this much, right now it feels really good and, if we decide not to go any further and just remain friends tomorrow, it still feels really good. I don't think anything but good can come from our knowing each other!"

"I don't know. This guy just sounds too good to be true. Where did you say you found him again…church? Let me just review my 'everything I ever wanted in a guy list.' Let's see, he's…" Naahhh, there's got to be something wrong with this guy. He just seems too perfect; like he just fell out of the sky or something. He sounds like everything you ever asked for…plus, he's got that whole Spiritual thing going on that's so important to you," my worldly friend said, snapping her fingers and leaning back in her chair, in envious laughter.

"Yeah," I thought, smiling to myself. "But I never would have been able to trust the possibility of love again, if it wasn't for my faith in God. I'm just letting God handle the details of my heart until I have to choose to receive love again, you know?"

"Yeah, choosing love, now that's what I'm talking about girlfriend…So tell me," she said, moving in closer, "How IS the sex?"

Smack—another thump from one girlfriend to the other.

"Ouch! What was that for? I just wanted the dirty details…Geeeez!"

Blushing, I replied, "Well, were not actually—you know—having sex right now."

"Oh, good for you girl, keep your relationship in line with God's will and watch Him bless the heck out of it," my Christian girlfriend said, tossing a piece of popcorn across the table while my other girlfriend sat there rubbing the sting from her arm.

"Yeah right, You're joking…You're not having sex…right," my worldly girlfriend laughed, as she continued rubbing on her arm and ducking popcorn. Then suddenly covering her mouth and sitting up straight she exclaimed,

"Oh my gosh, that's what's wrong with him isn't it? Oh, honey, I'm so sorry. I knew it was too good to be true, I just knew there was going to be something. Ohhhh, I just didn't know it would be…oh, honey," she said, reaching out as if to console me with one hand while the other continued to cover her mouth in disbelief.

"What? Huh? Noooo. Oh, Good heavens, No! There's absolutely nothing wrong with him like that!" I said, pulling her hand from her face. "He is more than okay in that department, for heaven's sake. We've just both made a mutual commitment to God that our desire is for the next one to be 'THE ONE,' and we both had made that choice about the same time in our lives so we've just agreed to not go there right now. That does not mean we don't want to, or that there is something wrong with either one of us! And that does not mean we are going to make it either…it's just that we are trying to live our lives in a way that would be pleasing to God, I guess. For heaven's sake. It's not that big a deal," I said, blushing and trying to change the subject.

"Nuh uhhhh," she said, laughing out loud and ducking the looming popcorn thrown from my Christian friend. "You are so not telling me you are acting like a virgin…are you girl?" she said giggling and slapping at the flying kernels. "Oh my gosh! You're serious, aren't you! No way!" she said, finally sitting up straight and searching my face for the truth. "No way! You cannot tell me you are that crazy about this guy and you don't want to make love to him? I mean, I know you're not a sex maniac or anything, but it's not like you've never had sex before. Why are you going all virgin all of a sudden? What's up with that?" she continued, letting the look on her face strike a chord in me that I was somehow living in delusion, or worse yet, that there was something wrong with me. "You are so not telling me that you are waiting until you get married to ever do it again…are you?" she offered, tilting her chin into her chest and looking at me with raised eyebrows, as popcorn fell from her hand.

"Now wait a minute," my other girlfriend interjected, as she opened her Bible and reached for a gulp of iced tea to wash back the little bits of popcorn that were stuck in her throat. "Your very life can become an expression of worship to God, when you are waiting on Him for stuff. It doesn't matter what you're waiting for. It even says so, right here in the Bible, if I can just find that darn passage," she continued, as she flipped the pages of her well-worn book.

"So you're really serious about this waiting thing, girlfriend? How come? I mean do you even…like…kiss and stuff?"

I responded by taking in a deep breath and rolling my eyes, "Yes, we kiss and stuff. I'm not saying I'm a saint, for heaven's sake. I didn't say I don't want to, and I'm certainly not saying it's easy, either. My goodness, I am human after all. But our small group and other friends have helped keep us accountable, because they are all supporting our decision. Everyone else in our group is doing the same thing. I mean, if what we were doing before wasn't working, what's wrong with trying it God's way and seeing what happens. I mean there are no guarantee that we are going to get extra blessings from God by denying ourselves, but if we do decide to terminate our relationship, it's going to be a whole lot easier to remain friends, and without having the chemistry of sex influencing our relationship, we are going to be a whole lot clearer about our choices. None of us wants to end up in divorce again! Anyways, the more I study God's word, the more it is becoming my CONVICTION, and not just some COMMITMENT. Who knows if I'll even ever get married again? All I am saying is it's my desire to try and live God's way, instead of my own."

As my Christian girlfriend winked at me over her reading glasses, flipping the pages of her Bible, I realized that I was now caught right in the middle of a conversation that may sound "too Christian" for my worldly girlfriend, and "not Christian enough" for my Christian friend.

"You know what? Whatever…to both of you," I said, holding up the palm of my hand. "I get the same response from my guy friends, too. As a matter of fact, I just got this email from a friend of mine who said that abstinence was not going to help build love, enhance my self worth, nor portray a more desirable picture of my virtue from a guy's point of view, and that men want to know what they are signing up for before they sign on! Oh, I could just spit, he made me so mad!"

"Oh, my gosh! What did you say?" my friend said, lowering her Bible to her lap to hear my response.

"Here, read what I wrote him back, for yourself," I said, reaching for the folded paper I had tucked into my purse.

I am not the person I was fifteen, five, or even two years ago—or for that matter, even yesterday. Why? Because of love, the entire lesson of it, the many contrasts of it. Want to know the most wonderful lesson I have learned about the kind of love God speaks of, and requires of me? It's that love is not optional. Yeah, it's actually a command—one given by the very God I serve. It's a choice and a commitment and—here is the big-gie—it's a CONDUCT! Yes, a conduct shown by our actions. Nothing I say, know, believe, give, or accomplish matters one little bit to God if I don't love Him with every part of me and let Him into every part of my life. And I am trying. I love God with all my heart, and because of that love I am making the effort toward a conduct that is glorifying to Him. I do it not to prove to you or the world that I am virtuous. It has nothing to do with a sense of self, but more to do with a desire to please heaven with actions that contradict the natural feelings and desires of the flesh. It's human nature for people (children, especially) to want and do what 'feels' good over what 'is' good for them. Learning love and living out mature acts of love takes emotional maturity (not necessarily chronological maturity, but in my case...). So, as far as sex—ahhh, sex—now, there is a feeling! Love, now, that elusive thing I have desired all my life, Love, is a choice. And I choose to love God with all of me. You, my friend—along with the rest of the world—you just get the reflection. If you don't like what you see, breaking the mirror won't make the image go away.

"Holy cow, girlfriend! Sounds like you need to get yourself a little sumpin' before you go and hurt somebody, if you know what I mean," my worldly girlfriend said, folding the printed paper back along its creased lines and sliding it across the table toward me with her eyebrows raised and chin tucked under once again.

"Hey, you know what, it's not just about me learning how to love the way I believe God intended. There are some fringe benefits to this abstinence stuff, too," I said, tossing the paper overhead into the wastebasket, "Ah—two points!"

"Nice shot, girl. So, like, what's the benefits?—'cause I ain't seein' no light at the end of that tunnel."

"Well, by my boyfriend sticking to his side of the commitment, when I get weak, knowing what I do to him when we are alone," I said winking, "I'm gaining a whole lot of confidence that he has what it takes to stick to his commitment to me in marriage—if we go there, that is. Not only that; by not having sex, I get the benefits of all the interesting things he has to come up with that sex would normally replace. It's really kind of romantic," I said, wondering if my friend was ever going to let up on me about the subject.

"Here it is!" my Christian girlfriend exclaimed, proudly, as she pointed to a highlighted passage she had written in her worn, leather Bible, "I knew I would find it," she said, reading aloud from her penciled notes in the margins.

"Look, I wrote these notes about waiting, right over Corinthians. 'Waiting forces us to slow down and notice what's going on around us and, perhaps, what others are going through. Our tendency is to compare ourselves with others. But, waiting can bring a different perspective into our lives, keeping us from making our problems bigger than they actually have to be. Waiting also allows God to direct our choices and make them clear," she said smugly, as she closed the text and placed her folded hands on top of the book. "I think it's great, what you guys are doing together, and I support you on whatever choices you and your honey make. Personally, I think you-know-who could learn a little something from you two!"

"Ugh—both of you are going to drive me insane!" I said, standing up to stretch my legs.

"You know what, girlfriend?" my worldly friend softened. "Whether the two of you end up married or not, in a way, I guess, I kind of envy you. It's really kind of romantic that you guys would do that for each other. You deserve the very best, and I'm really proud of you at least trying something to better your life and heal your heart. What you have been through, and how you are handling it…well, I guess if I really think about it, it makes some of the stuff I've been going through in my life seem a whole lot simpler," she said, offering me a hug.

"But I'm telling ya, right now," she asserted as she released me from her embrace, "I ain't about to give up sex for nobody! So, don't be sending none of your proper-datin'-ain't-nothing-happenin'-tonight-Christian-thinking-gonna-show-you-I-love-you-by-NOT-lovin'-ya guy friends 'round to knock on my front door, girlfriend! 'Cause that'd be like takin' candy from a baby!" she said, placing one hand on her hip, as the other hand plumped up her hair.

We all burst out laughing! You could have heard the snickers, snorts, and giggles for miles around. I found myself smiling as I realized that, although I may feel alien, at times, in both the Christian subcultures and worldly accepted cultures, the greatest moments of my life, as well as the strongest friendships, lay somewhere in the process of my defining my own relationship with God, while accepting the free will of those with whom I share my life's loving moments.

God was bridging the gap of understanding, once again, just as He has always done in my life, and I thought how very precious my girl-friends were to me, in the moments we shared Self♥Loving between us.

♥ A Fairytale Ending?

They say that a fairytale isn't a fairytale until you get to the final chapter. The tale, up to that point in the story, is largely full of twists and hairpin turns that can leave one breathless and even discouraged. One thing is for sure; wisdom doesn't come cheap, and finding gratitude from each lesson, each moment, and each chapter of my life, well, that requires a little patience. This chapter does not end in the typical fairytale finale for which most women swoon. No, the final chapter of my heart's tale has yet to be written, but this story and lesson in love does end on a richer and more Self♥Loving note than simply another ride off into the sunset.

I have become wiser in my understanding of love and Self♥Love, and recognized, early on in this romantic relationship, that there were major differences in our everyday lifestyles that, in the long run, would not sustain a marriage-bound commitment. I was able to keep the joys of this romantic tale in view, while taking in the essential moments necessary to see through to the truth. Self♥Love always demands the truth, and my final answer to his "Will You?" question, in the end, had to be a faith-filled, "No."

> ♥With each step forward in Self♥Loving, I become
> more effective in creating harmony for the final
> chapter of my heart's fairytale ending!

Today, as of the conclusion of this book, anyway, I find myself working at doing similar things as you are, right now: trying to accept each of life's beautiful lessons with enthusiasm and faith, and authentically living love. I have faith that God knows the desires of my heart, and that I will experience true love's kiss upon my lips before I take my last breath on this earth. Of that I am sure—unwearyingly, positively sure. Perhaps it has already been set in motion!

♥Waiting For Change?

I am sure each of us has experienced disappointments in our trust, and our investments into life, and, to the casual observer, some of my recipes might be construed as being delusional, arrogant, or even parochial. But whatever your view, know that my recipes, formulae, stories, and metaphors come from an impassioned belief that love does exist and is real, and that it ultimately comes from an intimate relationship with God.

So, if you've been waiting for something to change in your life, or if you're hurting, right now, and are looking for hope, I encourage you to take a "moment" to be honest with God about your feelings, and take "moments" with others to open yourself up to new possibilities.

If you have found this portion of the book to be inspirational in anyway, I invite you to personally tell four (yes, 4), friends about this book. By doing so, you will be planting four seeds of healing possibilities. Why am I asking you to tell four friends and not just one, two or three? That's a very good question so let me share a little story with you as it was once shared with me.

A Sower went out to plant the potential of healing among the land with four seeds in her pocket.

One of her seeds fell by the roadside, and was trampled underfoot, then eaten by the birds.

Another seed fell on rocky soil, and could not grow a root. At first, the Sower rejoiced at the sight of new growth, but, when the heat of day came upon the struggling plant, it withered and died.

Another of her seeds landed among the thorns. Once again, it began to grow, but as the new life started to shine, the thorns choked the life out of it- and it died, bearing nothing but weed. But the Sower did not become discouraged and she keep sowing.

Her final seed landed upon rich and fertile soil. It took root and bore fruit, 30, 60, and 100-fold! From that one little seed came hundreds of healing possibilities amongst the land.

Be a Sower of healing potential and SPREAD THE WORD! Thank you for allowing me to share some of my "moments" with you on this journey toward your own Self♥Loving.

> ♥ "I believe God wants to strengthen you, too. Let Him show you His love, and listen for His voice. He may just lead you to the specific ingredient that has been missing from your own Self♥Love Potions."

PART Two

Self-Help Work-Book Section

♥ Homework & Self♥ Love Work♥

We read to figure out what's going on around us, but we write to figure out what is going on inside of us. If we want to live in peace and contentment, we have to learn how to adapt our recipes. This is where you get to start working on your own Self♥Love Potions!

The following pages contain the basic outlines for some very fine recipes of Self♥Loving and learning. I have put them in the order discussed in the previous chapters of this book, with the first recipe being that of Spiritual awareness. I think it was Norman Vincent Peale who said, "Draw near to God and He will draw near to you."

Although I believe God never moves away from us, it can certainly seem as though God may be drawing nearer to our lives, as we actively move ourselves closer to Him, by seeking out His face within our everyday efforts and living. We all have to believe in something, but if what we believe in doesn't give us hope, peace of mind and contentment, I don't think we can create our best Self♥Love Potions recipes.

The following recipes can lead us closer to a place of hope, peace, and contentment as we begin with a recipe for building and acknowledging the healing power of faith. I believe eternal truth and the healing properties of Nature can and will change your life.

Self♥Love Potion Ingredient #1:

♥ Spirituality, the first ingredient.

> *Your personal connection to a higher
> power, the Spiritual aspect.*

♥ We don't always change because we see the light; sometimes it takes a little heat in the dark! Don't abandon your conscious choice to fate. Describe your personal relationship with a higher power.

♥ Since you were a child,

_____

_____

_____

♥ The voice you hear today,

_____

_____

_____

♥ Are you willing to do anything new today to see the rainbow? Invite "God" to speak to you? Ask? Search? Knock?

♥ (Suggestion: Don't go to scripture looking for *your* ideas, go searching for *God's*. If you don't know where to start, may I suggest you begin with the New Testament of the Bible. Get an inspirational version from the book store. Look for the truth, not the way you want to see it, but look for the truth, period. If you can't find it in the New Testament (for which I think there is substantial historical and documented evidence, as well as for the Christ it proclaims), but if you don't find it there, then I would encourage you to continue searching, always holding what you find up to the truth. Get a second and third opinion from different people before you make a decision.

~C

♥ Books I want to read: _____

_____

_____

Questions I want to ask: _____

_____

Groups I want to join: _____

_____

♥ People I want to get a second opinion from: _____

_____

♥ What I choose to believe today: _____

_____

~Listen, and you will hear .~

Self♥Love Potion Ingredient #2:

♥Accepting Responsibility.

♥Know Thyself. How well do you know yourself and how will you accept responsibility for your current situation right now?

♥List some truths about your life here: The good ones, and the not so pretty ones. Be honest with you. It's the only way to heal a weakness.

_____

_____

What might you choose to do differently now that you've identified the truths of your weaknesses? How will you approach this subject lovingly, if it involves others in your life?

_____

_____

Identify a list of things you desire to investigate further about yourself. Will you get some professional advice? If so, from where?

_____

_____

How might you find peace during change in your life?

_____

_____

Make a list of people whom you can count on for support to help you grow.

_____

_____

♥*Self-talk is very important. See yourself as worthy. You don't have to have a bad relationship to know you want a better one, which does not necessarily mean a "new one." Start with prayer and what you've already got, and be willing to accept responsibly for your healing and your pain.*~

Self♥Love Potion Ingredient #3:

♥ Letting Go of Envy.

> *Have you ever been jealous? Remember that things aren't always as they appear.

♥ Describe a situation you think this world (or God) is punishing you for?

_____

_____

♥ What might be a positive way of reviewing this situation, as you relate it to a loving lesson offered to you by your environment, releasing your negative perspective of it?

_____

_____

♥ Identifying your jealousy is the first step to letting go of it and letting God lead you to your true heart's desires. Describe some things you may be jealous or envious about. Are they similar to those situations you feel you are being punished for?

_____

_____

♥How might you find joy for those who possess the things you are wishing for?

_____

_____

~Think or feel about your life right now, using the view point that every-thing you have, everything you are and everything you do, is enough! Just do what you do and what you need will come. Does that change your self-picture? ~

Self♥Love Potion Ingredient #4:

♥Respecting the free will of others.

   ♥Accepting the free will of others with grace.

Choose Self♥Love by holding fast to your dreams while respecting the free will of others. Accept their free will choices with grace. It keeps the hardened reality of the world (a broken heart or lost hope) from destroying your identity and your view of life's true joys. Let others live with the consequences of their actions, and you live with yours. ~

♥Describe a situation in which you have tried to protect (or control) another person's free will.

_____

_____

♥What are some of the ways your attempts to protect or control another person accomplished your intentions?

_____

_____

♥What are the ways in which your attempts have been unsuccessful?

_____

_____

♥What have been the costs to you Emotionally, Physically, Financially, or Spiritually?

_____

_____

♥If you hadn't made those choices, where would the other person be now? Compare that to where you would be now.

_____

_____

♥How long do you want to continue this behavior, and what might be the possible rewards or risks of doing something different?

_____

_____

~ *Realize you are worthy of love not because of what you do, or give, or provide, but simply because of who you are. God's grace demonstrates that kind of love. We are all worthy of love. We just get side-tracked sometimes, trying to prove it to ourselves.* ~

Self♥Love Potion Ingredient #5:

♥*Listening .

> *Listen to what is really being said, and not just what you want to hear, then keep a clear perspective about the information being shared.

♥ Recall a conversation that may have been uncomfortable for you and list some of the words that caused a negative reaction in you.

_____

_____

♥ Using a thesaurus, list some alternative words which mean the same thing but are less tender to your ears. (You can share this list with your partner and friends.)

_____

_____

♥ After reconsidering the issue using your new list of words, decide if what you heard was really what was being said?? If not describe your assumptions, and the words that caused those assumptions.

_____

_____

_____

♥ Now, take your thoughts about your dilemma to a different place. You can ask your partner to go with you. Write down what you notice is different about the insight you get about the dilemma in these different places? Are you listening differently?

♥Go to the park, a place of worship, a coffee house, the kitchen table, the back yard, an ice cream shop etc…

_____

_____

_____

_____

_____

~For every word of criticism I gave (and there were lots) I tried to offer several more in encouragement.~

Self♥Love Potion Ingredient #6:

♥Journaling.

Journaling gives us clearer insight into to that which is important, but it takes time. Here's how to teach your brain to let it work for you.~

1. Find a quiet place. (I used to have to go into the bathroom—it was the only quiet place in the house!)
2. Bring a pen, paper, and a timer. Set the timer for ten minutes—no more the first time.
3. Just sit there. It's going to feel like a lifetime, and your mind will be racing with thoughts like, "*I am wasting my time. There are so many things I could be doing right now,*" but the trick is to just sit there for the full ten minutes.
4. Do this every night, adding one minute per evening, until you are up to a full thirty minutes. As you train your mind to realize you aren't going anywhere for a while, the pen will begin to glide across the paper. Don't judge what you're writing; just write. Thoughts, feelings, conversations, lists…anything…just write it!
5. If you find yourself writing about a dilemma, ask yourself the following questions:

How do you react to what your have read? If you found this piece of paper on the side of the road, what could you learn about the person who wrote it and what does the writer need to do or learn?

6. Over the following days, if you find yourself thinking about your dilemma, gently remind yourself you have plenty of time at the

end of the day to think about it, and get back to the matters you are working on at present.

At the end of each journaling session, decide what you want to do with what you wrote: destroy it? keep it? And how will you use this information?

Try it for the next seven days and see what happens.

Day One: Date_____

Set your timer and write whatever comes to mind:

_____
_____
_____
_____
_____
_____

♥Timer goes off: Now read it. What do you think or feel about what you are reading?

_____
_____

♥What can you be taught from, or learn about, the *person* who composed this information?

_____
_____

♥What do you think or feel the composer of the letter needs to do next and why?

~Journaling helps me get clarity from "Self♥Loving ♥Moments."~

Day Two: Date_____
♥ Set your timer and write whatever comes to mind:

_____
_____
_____
_____
_____
_____

♥ Timer goes off: Now read it. What do you think or feel about what you are reading?

What can you be taught from, or learn about, the *person* who composed this information?

What do you think or feel the composer of the letter needs to do next and why?

Day Three: Date_____
♥ Set your timer and write whatever comes to mind:

_____
_____
_____
_____
_____
_____

♥ Timer goes off: Now read it. What do you think or feel about what you are reading?

What can you be taught from, or learn about, the *person* who composed this information?

What do you think or feel the composer of the letter needs to do next and why?

Day Four: Date_____

♥Set your timer and write whatever comes to mind:

_____

_____

_____

_____

_____

_____

♥Timer goes off: Now read it. What do you think or feel about what you are reading?

What can you be taught from, or learn about, the *person* who composed this information?

What do you think or feel the composer of the letter needs to do next and why?

Day Five: Date_____

♥Set your timer and write whatever comes to mind:

_____

_____

_____

_____
_____
_____
_____

♥Timer goes off: Now read it. What do you think or feel about what you are reading?

What can you be taught from, or learn about, the *person* who composed this information?

What do you think or feel the composer of the letter needs to do next and why?

Day Six: Date_____

♥Set your timer and write whatever comes to mind:

_____
_____
_____
_____
_____
_____

♥Timer goes off: Now read it. What do you think or feel about what you are reading?

What can you be taught from, or learn about, the *person* who composed this information?

What do you think or feel the composer of the letter needs to do next and why?

Day Seven: Date_____

♥ Set your timer and write whatever comes to mind:

_____

_____

_____

_____

_____

_____

♥ Timer goes off: Now read it. What do you think or feel about what you are reading?

What can you be taught from, or learn about, the *person* who composed this information?

What do you think or feel the composer of the letter needs to do next and why?

Self♥Love Potion Ingredient #7:

♥ Identifying the many masks we live beneath.

Some of us have been wearing masks for so long that we have lost our-
selves in the expectations each one brings with it.
♥What is underneath?
List and explain in detail a few expectations from another person, or
from you, for a situation, relationship, job, household, friendship, etc.
Be as specific as you can.

_____

_____

_____

_____

_____

♥What are some ways in which your (or another's) expectations have
not been met? Are you hurt, angry, or numb as a result?

_____

_____

♥How many examples can you find in your daily (verbal or physical)
activities that might be masking those expectations from being understood by your partner?

_____

_____

♥Are you willing to share your list with your partner, child, friend, etc., and are you willing to authentically listen to a list provided by them? Write down some of your partner's expectations here. Do some of these expectations come as a surprise to you?

_____

_____

♥What are some possible ways in which you might respond differently, now that you and your partner's masks have been removed?

_____

_____

_____

_____

_____

~ The understanding of what faith can offer my life gives me courage to stand up for what I believe in and share that perception with others. ~

Self♥Love Potion Ingredient #8

♥Blessing yourself with a symbol of Self♥Loving.

♥ Perceptions♥ ~
Symbols allow us to take in a lot of information, put it into a neat package, and then manage it. When a police officer flashes his red lights, there is no need to explain who is in charge, where he gets his power, and what he wants. The symbol reveals it all. You can free yourself from negative reminders by turning them into symbols of Self♥Loving. ~
♥Make a list of some "things" that hold unhappy memories for you that you just can't seem to get rid of.

_____

_____

♥If you want to let go of the negative memories but keep the "things," what would be the best way for you to do that? Make a list of any positive feelings you might have toward these items.

_____

_____

♥What would it cost you to remodel, modernize, refashion, reconstruct, or revise these things so they become a symbol of hope, happiness, and growth? Create a plan, set a date, or hire a contractor. Whatever it takes to get you started. What is your first step going to be?

_____

_____

~ *It was a sparkling example that I was ready to let go of the pain and reclaim the positive, make amends for the harm I've done to myself esteem and create an inspiring foundation for my future.* ~

Self♥Love Potion Ingredient# 9

♥Asking for help.

♥ **Perceptions** ♥ ~

Many times, we think we have to handle our own problems independently (as if that were even possible to do) and we forget one very important thing: It's ok to ask for help. ~

♥Make a list of people you know who have had a dilemma similar to yours. You can even include people from history or fiction.

_____

_____

_____

_____

♥Ask at least three of these people for advice (or read a biography about them), and pay close attention to the techniques, tools, and wisdom they used to heal themselves. ♥What surprised you about their information, and how does it influence your thinking about your dilemma?

_____

_____

_____

_____

♥Do you think you can use any of their advice to modify your own behavior? If so, how?

_____

_____

_____

~ *"Just some food for thought, but you may be looking for the kind of help you require in the wrong place, and if you are, well, that might be the first thing you want to modify.*~

Self♥Love Potion Ingredient #10:

♥Learning from your pain, and sharing that healing with others.

♥Look at your life's struggles. What techniques did you use to help you at the time? List them here.

_____
_____
_____
_____
_____

♥What gifts might you choose to share with others, now that you've identified the gifts of your life's discomforts? How will you approach this subject? Write a book, start a club, offer your time? The possibilities are endless. List some ideas here:

_____
_____

♥Identify a list of people with whom you can identify, someone who may be going through a crisis that you have survived. Write their names and phone numbers here:

_____
_____
_____
_____
_____

♥ How might you find peace by offering your own personal encouragement during this time of change in someone else's life?

_____

_____

~*You've already got what someone else may need. Offer them a hand up, and you grow together. Take the next step and share your Self♥Love Potions with others.*~

Self♥Love Potion Ingredient #11

♥The Blending of romantic love and Self♥Love.

Two parts God's love (Self♥Love) to one part Romantic love.
♥What are you asking for in a partner?

_____

_____

♥Why are these things important to you?

_____

_____

♥Some important aspects of a loving relationship may be overlooked when we view them through romantic eyes only. On the following pages, there are some factors that are commonly accepted as being important in a healthy relationship. Rate your confidence that you and your partner can get along from 1-10. Then, substantiate your confidence or your concerns. (If you are not in a relationship, use this as an outline to illuminate what you might be looking for in a relationship.) If you find that you are uneasy about an area that is important to you, get it straightened out before making a serious commitment.

1. Spiritual Compatibility   Rating 1-10 _____
Clarification:

2. Life Purpose   Rating 1-10 _____
Clarification:

3. Chemistry   Rating 1-10 _____
Clarification:

4. Accepting Responsibility for own actions   Rating 1-10 _____

Clarification:

5. Respecting your opinions or your feelings. Which do you prefer? Why?
Rating 1-10 _____
Clarification:

6. Tolerating diversity between you   Rating 1-10 _____

Clarification:

7. Honesty   Rating 1-10 _____
Clarification:

8. Making and keeps commitments   Rating 1-10 _____
Clarification:

9.   Communicating thoughts and feelings   Rating1-10_____
Clarification:

10. Opinion and compatibility regarding:
Sex:

Children:

Drugs, Alcohol, Gambling:

Money:

Career:

Physical Health:

Family:

Holidays:

Don't assume that the romance will last forever, or that things will change for the better on their own. You have to mix the right ingredients together to get the desired results.

~♥~ Nutrition ~♥~

~My Nutritional Soap Box ~

Okay, today has been one of those days where I have spent the better part of the morning up on my nutritional soap box, after having spent the previous evening reading the book *Fast Food Nation* by Eric Schlosser.

So, here I am, standing at the front desk of my natural health care center's reception area, waving my pointing finger about, quoting all the reasons why fast food is so bad for our kids—how it makes them hyperactive with low test scores, etc. Now, it's time for lunch.

After spending a noble two hours at a Christian book store and walking out with more than a dozen books shoved into a plastic bag—all on the subject of self-control and following God's will for your life—I realize I've skipped lunch, and my stomach is about turn my head into a very large ache.

Next thing I know, I find myself pulling into the parking lot of Taco Bell. As I am walking across the cobblestone pathway toward the door, I think to myself, *I am a drone.*

This is exactly why these fast food establishments are so successful; because they market to people like me—who know better, but do it anyway.

As I am walking into this restaurant to order food that I know is not going to make me feel any better, I realize that I'm unwilling to go to the store and buy the live food that takes more time to prepare. Right then and there, I got it!

That's it, I thought.

Time. That's the key element. Time is really what these people are selling me. I'm trading some of mine for some of theirs. Only thing is, theirs is not going to offer my body any extra time on this earth, but I really don't want this headache I feel coming on, either. So, I order.

While the young man behind the counter is taking my order, he asks if I would like it with or without sour cream. And I'm smiling to myself, because I realize I ordered the chicken instead of the beef taco, and I'm feeling pretty good inside.

"That will be $1.79," he says, as I am drifting off toward the smell of coffee.

I'm thinking, *My time is probably worth $1.79,* as I plop it down on the counter.

Then I wonder how much time it would actually take me to go home and make an organic salad.

"Say, where is that smell coming from?" I ask, almost irritated as I look around the room. "I know that smell. That smells like Starbuck's!" I add, continuing to look for the coffeehouse logo I know so well.

"Yes ma'am, there's a coffeehouse right next door. Would you like anything else, ma'am," he asks again.

"Yeah. I'd like you to stop calling me ma'am, first of all, and no, thank you, that fresh chicken taco is going to be just fine," I say, rather flippantly.

He responds, with a wink, "Well, they're not actually fresh, ya know, ma'am," and smiles.

As I walk out the door, two Taco Supremes in hand (yes, the ones with sour cream), I pat myself on the back for not ordering a drink to go with it, even though I don't like the taste of soda anyway. So, with that feeling of elation, I proceed down the cement pathway and find myself standing inside Starbuck's coffeehouse. Now, mind you, it's about 100 degrees outside and I ask myself,

"Why am I standing inside a Starbuck's coffeehouse, about to order a hot coffee while holding a bag of tacos from Taco Bell?"

"May I help you?" a friendly voice asks from behind the counter.

"Uhhhh, huhhhhh," was all that came out of my mouth. Once all the marbles fell into place inside of my head, I said, "Yes, do you have anything cold, uhhh, that you can make with soy milk instead of regular milk? Oh, and no sugar, because that just makes me crazy. Oh, and can you make it without caffeine?"

Without blinking an eye he answered. "Yes ma'am. We can make you a decaf, soy latte over ice, if you like."

I fought the urge to tell him my preference on the usage of the word ma'am and instead, I quipped, "Great, I'll take it."

As I waited for my drink to be prepared, I justified my being there by looking for a birthday gift for my brother from amongst the shelves of cookies and coffee contraptions displayed conveniently in front of the order pick up line. Fortunately, I heeded the warnings from the little voice inside my head that was saying, *Put the cookies down and back away slowly.*

Once I got my iced soy decaf latte, tacos in hand, I made my way across the hot pavement to my car. As I slipped inside the leather interior, I realized leaving the top down on my car was probably not the smartest idea, but at this point my derriere was already neutralizing the seat temperature.

So there I sat, top down, keys in the ignition, air conditioner blowing, eating my Taco Supreme, and washing it back with my decaf latte, looking at the cover of one of the books I had just bought as it was peeking out from inside the plastic bag. The title: *Planning for Self-Control.*

As I watched the afternoon replay itself (as if projected on a movie screen in my head) I began to laugh out loud. I heard the words, *It is what you do that speaks so loudly that I can not hear your words.*

I think Buddha or some philosopher said it—I'm pretty sure I didn't just think it up. But, anyway, the point is I got the message!

If I desire to speak from an authentic position of inspiration I can't just quote words from atop my soap box and expect people to pursue those passions. I've got to tell the whole story as I live it!

> ♥I believe it's not the words that inspire people; people do…in their ordinary every day successes and failures.♥

To me, that's real life; one worth sharing and living with others. When it comes to nutrition, many of us are on the same page of confusion. There are so many books written on the subject that tell you, "Don't do this, but you have to do that," and they are all correct.

The key, when it comes to your diet, is finding what works for your lifestyle and just following a few simple guidelines during each season. I have discovered how to heal myself of the weaknesses I face, using Nature's dietary guidelines and some of Grandma's advice.

Over the next few pages, I want to share that information with you. I know that if I can do it, you can, too! Please keep in mind that this information should not be considered medical advice, and you should consult your doctor of health care before starting any new diet program or dramatically new health care regimen.

I'd like to go through the basics of each season and offer you some general information about each one. There are so many wonderful things that will never be done for you if you do not do them for yourself. These tiny moments can hold the choices you need to begin thinking, believing and practicing the healing power of enthusiastic faith and natural healing.

If we strive to eat the foods and colors of each season, I think we can be one step closer to meeting the chemical needs of our bodies. From there, we can choose how we want to support our weaknesses and enhance our strengths with other options. So, now is the time to start loving yourself on the inside and the outside, too.

As I drove back towards my office, I began the process of sorting through my thoughts about how I was going to offer the essentials of nutrition, from a more empathetic perspective. Pulling into the parking lot of my office, still deep in thought, I took a moment to freshen my lipstick in the rear-view mirror. As I wiped the remnants of sour cream from my chin, I smiled at the reflection as it reminded me to simply speak the truth in love.

Being human means being able to make poor choices followed by better ones. As we gather more empowering information, not only about the facts of nutrition, but about our own quality of life, we will become better equipped to balance the poor choices we make in our lives with the good ones. It's really pretty simple when you get right down to it.

So, let's get organized, so that we can eat right, exercise, pray, process, and, most importantly, enjoy the quality of our lives as we grow!

♥The Seasons♥
There are four seasons to a year,
For the purposes of
Cleansing, Resting, Building, and Playing.
We heal "one" year (four seasons) at a time.
Nature has a plan.

Look at the seasons, as expressed by a newborn baby, when cellular activity is at its highest peak.

Wake up from a nap: ♥Winter Rest
Want to eat: ♥Spring Building
Want to play: ♥Summer Expending
Dirty diaper: ♥Fall Cleansing
Back to sleep: ♥Winter Rest

♥On a cellular level, it takes an adult 365 days to do what a newborn does in just one! ♥

It takes time to heal, when you follow Nature's plan.

♥Fall

Fall begins September 21st and ends December 20th. Fall can sometimes leave me feeling "vapor-brained," or "just not feeling right," with no other physical symptoms to back up the unexplainable, unbalanced feelings, other than it's Nature's cleansing time of year. Fall is like being on the front line, emotionally speaking, and it's likely you'll get hit.

The emotional cleansing of Fall may even neutralize you, mix you up, and depress you, but if you give in to the cleansing feelings that may get kicked up during this time of year, it's because you've made a choice to do so. Even if you become fatigued, frustrated, or scared to death during a Fall cleansing, you CAN still choose not to be discouraged. This cleansing will pass! It may last a day, a week, or several. It just depends on how aware you are of the process and what you do to support yourself during the Fall cleanse.

Some people actually enjoy the cleansing process of Fall, because of the rewards that are found on the other side of the healing crisis. (See "healing crisis" for more information on this incredible gift of healing.)

For emotional support you may want to explore journaling. Keep a notepad next to your bed, or in your purse or car, so you can write out random thoughts and organize them. You can turn to Self♥Love Potion #6 for more information about this powerful healing tool.

A great exercise for clear thinking is breathing. No, really. I'm serious. Ten deep breaths in a row, three times throughout the day. Breathe deeply in for one count, hold for four counts then push the air out for two forceful counts. It really works!

To make the transition into Fall gracefully, be sure to eat lots of orange and brown colors: squash, pumpkin, eggplants, and lots of veggies. As always, green leafy vegetables are important. If you have joint pain during this time of year, I have found MSM, 1gram per 50lbs body-weight, twice a day, to work wonders on my poor little joints. I've also added Glucosamine, two tablets twice a day; liquid minerals, 1oz in the morning, and massaged my joints with Wintergreen or Birch oil.

Since this is the cleansing time of year, I like to do a Tiao-He Cleanse for ten days, some time between September and mid-November. I get my products from Nature's Sunshine. I've listed their number in the back of this book for your convenience. (Please consult a medical professional before adding any supplements to your own routine.)

I love aromatherapy oils, and some of my favorite smells during this time of year are Cinnamon, Apple, and Spruce. Spruce is probably the most healing oil for me during Fall. This oil grounds the body's energy and opens emotional blocks, for balance. Historically, the Lakota Indians used it to enhance their communication with "the Great Spirit." As a child, my grandma used to put a drop of the essential oil over my temples and heart, and on my feet to stimulate my immune system. She said that Nature used these plants to restore energy and rejuvenate the wild animals that slept beneath these trees at night. It's funny how I feel the same way after putting this oil on my feet at night during Fall.

Difficulty making simple decisions, compulsive behavior—even obsessing—can be a sign that the Fall cleansing process is in full swing. If I find myself feeling like this any other time of the year, it's usually due to stress, and I will make adjustments in my diet or social schedules to compensate. But during the Fall I try to just let my body and emotions run their course.

It's not uncommon to hear people say, "I have never really felt the same after…(some nerve-racking event)." Even if the stress was a positive stress, it can still be harmful to the body. Keith Smith (a Master Herbalist in Escondido, and former teacher of mine) taught me the following herbal recipe, and I use it whenever I just don't feel right. The results are dramatic. Actually, you may feel worse for the first week or two, as the body reorganizes itself. How long it takes to rebalance your-self depends on how long you have been out of balance in the first place.

Also, keep in mind that (according to Keith) couples tend to get stressed together, with one partner initially drawing on the other's energy so much they both become depleted—what Keith calls "switched" or "reversed polarity." Based upon his own observation, he believes that being in a state of reversed polarity for more than six years sets the stage for autoimmune disorders.

♥The Recipe:

The four herbs Keith believes work together to rebalance the nervous system, nourish the body, and gently encourage the body to switch back to normal polarity are:

IMMC: a Chinese formula to generate Chi in the body

THIMJ: traditionally used to support the thyroid and glandular sys-tem (where we hold emotional energy)

Spirulina (my favorite herb): 72% protein;

RNA & DNA positive food containing all your essential amino acids, B-Complex vitamins, and a variety of minerals.

Valerian Root, St. John's Wort, or some other nervien. These help nourish the nervous system while building emotional strength. If you are already taking any kind of prescription nervien, anxiety, or blood pressure medications, you should not use these over the counter nerviens in conjunction with them. Again, a word of caution, please get medical advice before taking any supplements.

I use liquid minerals and/or a lower bowel stimulant, like LBSII, when I need to help my body expel toxins on its own terms, as well.

Keith was always sure to remind me to take my herbs faithfully, not drink caffeine (yeah, right), and try to rest. Instead of my normal work-out routine, I have to do light exercise during this time period so my body can use its newfound energy to swing back into action!

Most often it's the type "A" personalities; you know, the ones who are bright and accomplishment-oriented (*smile*–who me?) that just won't rest or give up the caffeine, and then become energetically unbalanced. The psycho-Spiritual lessons that come from being out of balance are generally ones of letting go and surrendering control. The lesson is to reprioritize your life.

♥ Winter

Winter starts December 21st and lasts through March 20th. It's Nature's time of rest and recovery. This is the healing time of year when Nature goes into hibernation and prepares for Spring building. I call Winter the transition time of year—a time to go within and let Nature reveal the morals to all bedtime stories of the past year.

I like to take a fifteen-day "Stress Pack"—high in vitamins and minerals—sometime between Mid- December and mid-March. I use food enzymes with all meals of substance during these months as well, because my meals tend to be heartier.

Winter is the time to eat barley and seeds like sunflower, sesame, and pumpkin. These are warming foods that heat up the body. Also, look for foods like cereals, grains, brown rice, wheat germ, and oats.

Good foods for Autumn and Winter menus should include apples, pears, bananas, dates, celery stalks, kiwis, oranges grapefruits, tangelos, concord grapes, persimmons, tomatoes, avocados, Romaine lettuce, potatoes, pineapple, sweet potatoes, butter lettuce, cauliflower, yams, bell peppers, pecans, filberts, and carrots. Always eat your green, leafy vegetables to help with elimination of higher fat foods during this time of year.

As for essential oils, I love the oils of Humility, Harmony, Valor, and Joy. These are all combination oils from a company called Young Living (Y.L.). I love Y.L. combination oils because they blended so beautifully, and I don't have to do the hard work of mixing and matching. I can just reach for the one I want and rub them right on to the bottoms of my feet. I take them with me when I go for a massage as well.

Winter is a time to nurture and spoil myself. I love to cozy up with friends and make great Winter memories! I like to use lots of lavender in my Winter sea salt bath soaks and try to take a time out at least twice a week for this cleansing ritual during the Winter months.

I incorporate lots of prayer time, guided imagery, and personal meditation time into my daily routine during Winter, as well, since this is a time of year to enjoy the tranquility of the clean spaces we've created in our bodies.

♥Spring

I think the key to a fabulous Summer lies in the *Spring building*. Spring is a busy birthing time for Nature. If you've never taken the time to plan for your total health, Spring is the time to do it. You must see yourself as a lovable soul, true, but that loveable soul is living within a vessel that needs your constant attention, if it is to think, feel, and do its best, as well as attract likewise in your life.

Let's face it, our bodies play a large part in attracting the man (or woman) of our Springs! If you don't have a plan for your body, Spring is the perfect time to build one. It's a time to tune in and tune up your body, otherwise, you may end up showing off more of that fabulous flab than you were prepared to, come Summer!

You will probably find yourself naturally inclined to work on your appearance and the building of your total outward package during Springtime, anyway, because Nature naturally tends to turn up the chemistry a notch or two during this seasonal cycle. And, ladies, men still tend to pursue with their eyes first, chemistry or not. So, plan what you want to convey with that attractive, physical package, and Spring will help you out in the chemistry department.

Since Spring is a time for building and revitalizing, it makes sense that it would be a time of year when Mother Nature pulls the minerals and nutrients from the ground to nourish the next generation of seeds. It's the time of year when the law of natural selection is at its highest peak.

After three Fall months of cleansing and three Winter months of resting, you should be looking your best now! You won't want to take away from protein storage by skipping meals, because your oxytocin levels (love-sick levels) are at their highest peak right now.

Use a protein supplement or slip a protein bar into your purse, so your body doesn't starve itself. I don't care if you're hungry or not, you gotta have a little food in your stomach to keep your body from thinking it's starving. Once your body thinks it's starving, it will start taking the protein out of the toned muscles you are trying to put on your curves and your muscles will begin to drape your bones rather than shape them. So, keep a little something in your purse for in between or skipped meals.

My mentor and dear friend, the late Dr. Bernard Jensen, would tell me that juice therapy worked very well during Spring. He said that optimal tissue healing would come about within the body, partially due to the naturally high amounts of energy in the foods and sprouts during this time of year.

My grandma would tell me that the stalks of most vegetables are highest in nutrients during this time of the year, as well. Most of her Spring recipes were made of foods plucked fresh from her garden. Oh, the salads she would make!

She told me that the word "salad" comes from the Latin word "sal," meaning "salt." I guess Caesar used to put salt all over his Spring veggies, and next thing you know—bingo—salad was invented. I think it was the Egyptians, though, that cornered the market of mixing oil and vinegar with oriental spices. When they started pouring them over their greens, that's where we had the salads that more closely resemble the kind of Spring greens we eat today.

Spring is the time of year to select the best of the garden greens for your family meal, and it's just what the herbalist ordered. Greens have a tendency to neutralize acid in our bodies, and an alkaline environment is what the mind prefers. So, if you can't get enough greens in your diet by eating them, do what I do and cheat with NSP's "Greenzone."

Greenzone is a combination of greens that you mix in water. Not my favorite tasting drink in the world, but at least I know I'm getting my daily dose of greens when I just can't seem to get them in my normal diet.

Absorb the nutrients from Spring's leafy plants, and I'll bet you will have more than enough energy to expend in the burning Summer months ahead!

Spring and Summer Menus should include: strawberries, cantaloupe, cherries, apricots, watermelon, peaches, nectarines, honeydew, melon, plums, Crenshaw melons, canary melon, fresh figs, bananas, tomatoes, romaine lettuce, broccoli, almonds, spinach, red leaf (all leaf)lettuce and all the greens you can get your hands on!

♥ Summer

Summer officially begins June 21ˢᵗ, the day the sun is at its northern-most position relative to earth. It's the longest day of light of the year. I had a friend ask me once why it felt like Nature was stretching the sunsets out over a longer period of time, during the evening hours between the seasons of Spring and Summer.

My flip and teasing answer was that God knew we needed more daylight in order to see through the combustible energy-blindness Summer unleashed between man and woman during that time of year.

Actually, according to Pat Palmer, professor of astronomy at the University of Chicago:

> *The sun's gravitational pull creates a slingshot effect, accelerating the earth through a hairpin turn just before Summer. At that time, the earth is moving fastest past the sun, spinning on its axis in the same direction it orbits (counterclockwise), meaning your home must rotate about 361 degrees to face back at the sun. That extra degree makes solar noon (when the sun is directly overhead) occur later each day. Visualize sunrise taking one step forward into day and sunset taking one step forward into night.*

Professor Palmer calls it "a simple case of astronomical attraction and declination."

A perfect explanation for my earlier dating life!

Summer is just kinda that way. It's a very high vibration time of year. Nature pours forth her abundance, and it's a time when we want to utilize our newly built muscles on energy projects and vacations. It's the time to express yourself, but watch that tongue during the fiery

Summer months, because, although Summer gives its energy to expression and speech, you're responsible for the words!

Summer energy governs the intuition and the heart (oh, big revelation there)! Did you know that the heart pumps over 3,000 gallons of blood per day to the lungs! I sure am glad the heart doesn't complain about how much energy it has to put into to each and every pump!

Professor Jack Worsley, a noted teacher of acupuncture, describes the small intestines as *"the separator of the pure from the impure"*—kind of like sorting out and extracting the good from the bad of what we take in, whether it's food, thought, emotion or action.

You will probably eat lighter and look for cooler foods, like salad and fish. I try not to eat past sunset. It's just better for digestion. But remember, sunset will get later and later into the evening as Summer moves on, so keep your eye on the clock. Six o'clock is the normal cut off for dinner time, but during Summer, I'll go as late as eight, nine, or even ten o'clock, depending on how late I'll be staying up. The later the meal, the lighter I go.

I believe that if an organ of the body is unbalanced or overstressed in its season, you will probably experience the expression of it in the following season. Summer is not the time you are going to want to eat a lot of fried foods and milk products. Things like salt, animal organs, sugar, refined processed foods and caffeine should be limited or eliminated during these months, depending on how healthy you are going into Summer in the first place.

Nature's timing is perfect with providing us many wet and cooling foods. My rule of thumb: eat the foods of the season because Nature has a reason!

Emotionally speaking, Summer is a time to receive: grounding, success, individuality, stability, security, health, courage, positive emotions, desire, pleasure, passionate love, change, movement, assimilation of new ideas, family tolerance, surrender, working harmoniously and creatively with others, and everything related to the material world. To do this, you have to release: self-centered thinking, insecurity, violence, greed, anger, purposelessness, jealousy, envy, and the desire to possess.

I like to use the essential oils of lemon, orange, tangerine, apple, and lavender. Be careful in the sun though, because some of these oils can create a photosensitive reaction in the sun.

The fruits of your Spring labor (planning and building) should be paying off by Summer! Remember, fruits stir things up in the body, and your activity level should use up the sugar from the fruits you're craving. The season's fruits are easier to get in abundance, so I have to make an effort take as many greens as possible, because, although fruits stir it up, ya gotta have the greens to carry things out of the body.

Try a banana smoothie for breakfast instead of that banana waffle. Add one extra serving of vegetables to your dinner in place of dessert just once or twice this week. Don't like veggies? Try that green drink I was telling you about, mixed with water, once a day, instead. Don't like exercising either? Try walking to the corner video store instead of driving.

Over the hot Summer months, these activities will add up to a HOT Summer you! Some of the things I do almost ritualistically during the hot Summer months is take my colloidal minerals, 1oz every morning, because my body is going to be staying up and out later, and using more energy.

Minerals are like the sparkplugs of the body. For the hotter Summer days when I'm perspiring more, I'll even throw a scoop of "Recovery," from NSP, in my water bottle. It helps optimize recovery and minimize fatigue, and helps me stay hydrated. During Summer, it's more important than ever to drink your water.

♥Water

Although water is not technically considered a nutrient, it's one of the most powerful and healing substances we can put into our bodies. We could probably survive without food for several weeks, but without water we would only survive a few days.

Water keeps us from poisoning ourselves with waste products and toxins that are by-products of our own metabolism. Water is important, no matter what the season, but the soaring temperatures of the hot Summer months make it even more vital.

Most tap water is full of chloride, fluoride, and who knows what else, so I suggest you drink Spring or purified water. One of the things I like to do with my drinking water is pour it into a big glass container and leave it out on my patio in full sun for three or four days. It soaks up all the sun's energy and removes some of the chlorine as well. On less than sunny days, you can just boil the heck out of the water for about five to ten minutes. That reminds me of a joke.

How does a priest make holy water?

Answer: He boils the hell out of it! Ha ha!

Did you know that if you want to lose a few pounds you simply need to drink more water! If the body doesn't get enough water, it has trouble metabolizing the fat, and you end up with poor digestion, increased toxicity, and water retention. Water carries nutrients and oxygen to cells through the blood and regulates our body temperature when we perspire. It also helps lubricate joints, and helps us breathe by moistening lungs, making it easier to intake oxygen and release carbon dioxide.

Did you know you lose a pint of liquid each day just from breathing out? So, how much water do you need? One rule of thumb is one-half your body weight in ounces, *daily*. Overweight people should drink an extra 8 oz glass of water for every 25lbs they're overweight and spread the water intake throughout the day. Beer, coffee, tea, and carbonated and sweetened drinks contain lots of stuff that's not healthy, and should not be considered water substitutes.

I pulled the following information about water off the Internet; the author is unknown to me, but the information is worth investigating:

> 75% of Americans are chronically dehydrated. In 37% of Americans, the thirst mechanism is so weak that it is often mistaken for hunger. Even MILD dehydration will slow down one's metabolism as much as 3%.
>
> One glass of water shut down midnight hunger pangs for almost 100% of the dieters studied in a U-Washington study. Lack of water is also the #1 trigger of daytime fatigue. Preliminary research indicates that eight to ten glasses of water a day could significantly ease back and joint pain for up to 80% of sufferers.
>
> A mere 2% drop in body water can trigger fuzzy short-term memory, trouble with basic math, and difficulty focusing on the computer screen or on a printed page.
>
> Drinking five glasses of water daily decreases the risk of colon cancer by 45%, plus it can slash the risk of breast cancer by 79%, bladder cancer by 50%.

Are you drinking the amount of water you should every day?

♥Channels of Elimination & the Healing Crisis.

The American Cancer Society has said that it takes as long as twenty years to develop cancer. Symptom-suppressing drugs can even compound the problems because they can drive the basic cause deeper into the tissues.

Have you ever heard of the term "healing crisis?" If your answer is no, then you may have a difficult time understanding what I am about to share with you. Natural healing actually requires us to experience some of the symptoms we might consider illness on our way toward healing. Yes, that's what I said; healing actually requires our bodies to expel toxins which may in fact feel like illness.

To rid the body of toxins, you have to stir them up to get them to come out. The body will generally move toxins out of the system though one of the four major channels of elimination. Those channels are the bowel, the bronchial tubes (lung structure), the kidneys, and the skin.

If you look at the obituaries, no matter what the disease is, you will find that the death is going to be because of a kidney failure, pneumonia, or bronchial tube, lung, or bowel failure.

See, the bowel wall is made up of a second-rate tissue in respect to getting rid of toxic material from the body. In other words, it is very slow in transit time and when we are stressed and tired, the bowel works even more slowly.

When toxic materials are left in the body, they will settle in the weakest areas, while the other channels of elimination try to carry those toxins out of the system.

You will probably find that most natural healers will guide your nutritional suggestions toward taking care of these four elimination channels first, since the backup and settling of these toxins in our bodies is what causes most of our physical problems in the first place.

European Homeopath Constantine Herings states, "All cure comes from within out, from the head down, and in the reverse order as the symptoms have appeared in the body."

Simply stated, starting from where you are now, you will relive past troubles, pain or sickness as you undergo the reversal process of healing and your body tries to carry toxins out of the body.

Once you begin to change toward the positive in any area of your life, you're going to be kicking up old stuff. It will generally take the four seasons to heal one layer of tissue during this time, during the reversal of the course of disease, you are going to experience what we call "the healing crisis."

This crisis is the natural means the body uses to get rid of the toxins that can be harmful to the body's tissues before the body begins to heal those tissues. The most recent symptoms are always experienced first.

If the body has been so weakened by the long term effects of nutritional deficiencies and toxic build up, a person can actually make themselves weaker by trying to do too much healing or cleansing too fast.

Natural healing takes time. We don't get sick in one day, so even if you want to, you're not going to get healthier in one day, either…even if you feel like it! I always laugh when someone calls me on the phone with words of praise and elation over how wonderful they are feeling, two or three days after trying a new Self♥Love Potion. I simply smile to myself and say: *Thank you for your kind words, and I hope you will write down how wonderful you are feeling.*

They will ask me why I want them to write it down and I simply respond by saying it's just good to keep a record of their progress. But in reality, I know that if they have had years of nutritional neglect, then suddenly feel that good, they are just about to enter into the healing crisis.

In other words, the body will use all that newfound energy and put it to work getting out the toxins, so the body can return to that kind of positive state, permanently. If you do too much cleansing or healing too fast, you run the risk of landing yourself smack dab in the middle of a healing crisis that is going to feel just like the illness you're trying to get over, and this is why many people will give up just before they get the best results from their efforts.

My suggestion is that you start slow, remain consistent, and embrace each healing crisis as a sign that your body still has a little fight left in it!

Dr. Henry Lindlahr said, *"Give me a healing crisis and I will cure any disease."*

Hippocrates, the Father of Medicine, said, *"Give me a fever and I will cure any disease."*

The question now is; What do YOU say?

♥ So how do you know? ♥

So, how do you know the difference between a healing crisis and illness? That is the question I get a lot, especially from allopathic professionals.

> ♥I like to refer to the healing crisis as the exception to the rule, and illness as sort of a long, drawn-out syndrome of symptoms. ♥

You must be the judge as to what threat your health may be in, and I highly recommend you get professional advice whenever you are in doubt. But ask yourself this question to help you decide. Had you been doing something better or worse for your body, mind, or Spirit just before the illness hit? If the answer is "better" and then suddenly you started feeling a little sick, then chances are you're having a healing crisis, and you need to let it run its course without suppressing the channels of elimination.

Generally, a healing crisis takes less time to express itself than the original illness, and you feel much lighter, healthier and clearer once you get to the other side of the crisis.

Illness, however, is just the opposite. In a book written by Blair Justice in 1988, entitled *Who gets Sick?*, she writes:

> Disease is not so much the effect of noxious external forces—the bugs, both literal and figurative, in our lives—as it is the faulty efforts of our minds and bodies to deal with them. Most of the bugs, the literal kind, already reside in our bodies. When our responses to problems in life are excessive or deficient, the central nervous system and hormones act on our immune defenses in such a way that the microbes aid and abet disease.

Deepak Chopra, M.D, in his 1989 book entitled *Quantum Healing*, writes:

> If we find diseases in our body, they are there because we've created an environment that supports them. At the very instant that you think, 'I am happy,' a chemical messenger translates your emotion, which has no solid existence whatever in the material world, into a bit of matter so perfectly attuned to your desire that literally every cell in your body learns of your happiness and joins in.

A reporter from *Energy Times* told me she was writing an article on colds and flu and wanted my opinion as to why medical science has not been able to cure these pesky seasonal nuisances? My answer? Well, I believe that if we were ever able to cure the common cold, we would kill the human species.

My opinion is that these, sometimes twice yearly, symptoms are the cure to so many other diseases. It's the way the body naturally moves out the mucous, toxins and poisons in our systems to make room for healthy tissue growth.

When we are babies, our immune systems are provided with a number of opportunities, from teething to normal childhood diseases, to learn how to activate the immune response and respond to a viral or bacterial invader. However, in our "pink pill for a morning headache" and "blue pill for an evening headache" world, the first thing TV teaches us to do when we have a runny nose or a cough is to take a pill to stop the catarrhal or mucus.

New mothers are being sent home from the hospital with a bag full of company incentives to buy their products for fever, cough, and cold remedies for their newborn babies.

> ♥What we must ask ourselves is, does this way of
> suppressing and driving the inflammation
> back into the body make us healthier or weaker? ♥

By preventing toxins from being expelled, are we just stacking the deck in favor of disease? Are we really born with a cough syrup or aspirin deficiency? I don't think so. Although heredity does play an important role in how disease develops through out your life, you are responsible for your health and have a lot more control than you can imagine.

If you live your life in a way that encourages disease, blocks the channels of elimination, under-nourishes the body, and stresses the heart and mind, heredity will decide which form your particular illness is going to take.

Health is so much more than being drugged up, symptom free, suppressed, and subdued. True health requires us to allow the body to do exactly what is has to do to survive the lifestyle we have chosen to live.

Dr. M. Ted Morter, Jr. states, in his 1995 book entitled *Your Health Your Choice,*

> The body is a self-healing, self regulating, unified creation that never makes a mistake. The power that built the body from a single fertilized egg doesn't suddenly turn off at birth. Everything the body does is completely logical.

Did you know that it is perfectly natural for a person to have catarrh (or mucous) to excess whenever any of the elimination channels are not working properly?

The term catarrh comes from the Greek words *cata* (down) and *rhein* (flow), meaning to 'flow down,' and it refers to the mucus produced due to tissue inflammation. Catarrh precedes the onset of any disease and is a universal symptom. It is also a condition that people can take care of by themselves.

Acidity and catarrh appear during any elimination process. Which is why it's so important to keep those channels of elimination open when we are trying to heal.

Catarrh can developed when the kidneys are not working well, when the skin is not eliminating to its fullest potential, when the bronchial tract and lung structure are loaded and not expelling efficiently, and especially when the bowel is not moving along as fast as it should. The lymphatic system is also involved in the elimination of catarrh, and it is through the lymphatic system that catarrh is delivered to other parts of the body.

According to the late Dr. Bernard Jensen:

> If elimination is impeded, the catarrh may be forced to settle in the weakest organs of the body, creating conditions we have come to name as disease. When the body becomes well-saturated with the acid poisons resulting from faulty food, a person can suffer from one or more of the many catarrhal disorders.

We can call these catarrhal disorders by many names, and I have listed some of them here for your further investigation:

Catarrh of the stomach called gastritis, Catarrh of the mouth called stomatitis, Catarrh of the throat called diphtheritis (diphtheria), Catarrh of the nose called rhinitis, Catarrh of the bronchi called bronchitis (hay fever, asthma, etc.), lungs called pulmonitis (influenza, pneumonia,), the eyes called conjunctivitis (trachoma), the ears called otitis, the brain called phrenitis, also meningitis, of the small intestine called enteritis, of the large intestine called colitis, of the appendix called appendicitis, of the liver called hepatitis, of the pancreas called pancreatitis, of the kidneys called nephritis (Bright's disease), of the vagina called vaginitis (leukorrhea).

While far from being complete, the above list offers us an interesting view of how the body can take one harmful habit and, slowly but surely, create a chronic condition that finally affects every organ, structure, and function in the body.

♥The Basics♥

So, what are some basic things you can do to begin opening up those channels of elimination to allow the body to eliminate those toxins? Let's take a closer look at those systems before we go any further.

♥The Colon:

The colon affects the entire body. Most Naturopaths feel that a bowel elimination after each major meal is important. Yes, I said after every major meal! Many medical doctors will tell you a bowel movement every 2-3 days is perfectly acceptable, but does that mean it's healthy? NO!

Constipation contributes to the lowering of our immune resistance, predisposing us to illnesses and the degenerative chronic process. It increases the workload of the other eliminative organs—kidney, skin, liver, lungs, and lymph. As toxins accumulate in the tissues, digestion then becomes poor, and partially digested material further prevents the building of good, healthy tissue. Have you ever heard of the term "autointoxication?" It is when the body literally poisons itself to death by maintaining a cesspool of decaying matter in the colon.

Fluids taken into the body are absorbed into the bloodstream through the walls of the colon, affecting every major organ in the body. Skin eruptions, mucous buildup, and kidney problems are just a few examples of the colon's reflex action. Autointoxication can be a causative factor for almost any disease.

A great book to read is *Tissue Cleansing through Bowel Management*, by Bernard Jensen. It's a wonderful book filled with interesting suggestions on colon cleansing, and I think it's worth investigating.

♥The Lungs

The lungs are very sensitive structures. If they are unable to efficiently blow off carbon dioxide, carbonic acid is formed in the body and this will stress the kidneys' as well as the heart's activity. Obviously, you want to pass on smoking, but did you know that daily aerobic exercise and deep breathing could strengthen lung tissue, as well as oxygenate the system, too?

Traditionally speaking, the single herbs of Marshmallow, Fenugreek, Mullein, Comfrey, and Slippery Elm have all been used to strengthen and cleanse the lungs. I have even heard that locally grown Bee Pollen has been reported to alleviate allergy symptoms.

As I mentioned earlier, cleansing the colon helps take the stress off the lungs, and dry skin brushing helps, too. We will talk more about that in a moment.

Emotionally speaking, I have found those with chronic lung weakness tend to resist breathing in life to the fullest. Here we must affirm the faith to look beyond the appearance of lack and see a neverending supply of hope and Spirit.

Journaling can help to reverse old mental patterns. I like to diffuse Eucalyptus, Cypress, Sage, and Sandalwood essential oils to help stimulate and clear the lungs of mucous.

♥The Kidneys

According to ancient Chinese philosophy, fear has long been associated with bladder and kidney problems. If the kidneys become so stressed that they start producing ammonia, it can go to the brain. This would not be a good thing! You can die from that kind of body reaction.

We need to keep water flowing freely through the body to flush the kidneys. A half ounce of fluid for each pound of body weight is considered the basic amount of water needed by the body to keep the bladder and kidneys functioning properly.

Single herbs like Chamomile, Parsley, Uva ursi, and Cornsilk, as well as Vitamin B-6, have been used historically to support kidney and bladder function and deal with problems of water retention, incontinence, and frequent or painful urination. Chiropractic adjustments have worked wonders, as well.

My grandma would place me in a warm bath of rosemary to help ease the discomfort of a bladder infection. She would also rub juniper and Eucalyptus over the bottom of my feet.

♥The Skin

The skin is the largest organ of the body and controls our temperature by opening its pores to allow perspiration to cool us, or closing them to maintain our body temperature. It is also involved in respiration. Yup, I did say respiration.

The skin actually needs to breathe to be healthy! If you have skin problems, I have found it's usually due to the other organs of elimination being over stressed or backed up (as well as hormones imbalances to). But, if the body is not eliminating toxins efficiently, lots of other, seemingly unrelated problems pop up.

Keep those other channels open and moving. Exercise not only increases circulation to all parts of the body, but it makes you sweat, and that helps the skin, especially. Natural fiber clothing (wools, cottons, silk, etc.) allows the skin to breathe freely, while synthetics (nylon, polyester) prevent your skin from breathing. I just hate nylons!

Did you know that you should eliminate two pounds of waste acids daily through your skin? Good thing new skin is formed every twenty-four hours! Dry skin brushing is one of my favorite things to suggest for the skin. It really helps the skin to shed its dead cells and eliminate uric acid crystals, catarrh, and other acids in the body.

Use a softer brush if you are going to do your face. You can pay BIG bucks to have a professional exfoliation done to your face, but a dry skin brush costs only a few dollars, and you can do your entire body with it. Dry skin brushing is really easy to do, and it leaves your skin feeling soft as a baby's butt!

To dry skin brush, all you need is a dry vegetable-bristle brush. Nylon will just rip the skin to shreds. Start at the bottom of your feet and brush toward your head, covering the whole body, except the face. When you get to the face, use a gentler motion. Brushing before you take a bath will loosen the dead skin cells so that they can be washed away. It also increases the circulation to the skin. Do it daily.

I suggest that you use only pure soap and natural creams, cleansers, and lotions on your skin. If you want to try an interesting experiment, rub some garlic on the bottom of your feet. You should taste it in your mouth within just a few minutes! That's how fast the circulatory system can pick up and distribute to the rest of your body whatever you put on your skin! It's amazing.

In the next section, I have given you some great natural recipes for lotions and creams. I like to go to the mall and pick up a great smelling bottle of this or that, just like anybody, but for my regular daily routines I like to stick to the potions I can make in my own kitchen.

We have to watch the caffeine, chocolate and sugar intake, because they can rob the system of Complex Bs, which play a big part in tissue integrity. The single herbs of Burdock and Yellow dock have traditionally been used to cleanse the blood and, in so doing, assist the skin directly.

♥ Some Basic Dos and Don'ts ♥

Now that we know a little more about the four main channels of elimination, let's look at the following list of dos and don'ts, and simply pick one or two things, starting this week, or even this month, and begin to eliminate them over the next few seasons.

Things you may want to consider reducing or eliminating are red meats (beef and pork), white sugar, white flour, white bread, prepared cereals, processed and preserved foods, canned fluids with meals, pop, coffee, black tea, alcohol, table salt, black pepper, cow's milk products, and pasteurized and preserved foods.

Now think about replacing them with fish and fowl, honey, maple syrup, fresh, stone-ground whole wheat flour, whole-grain breads, cooked whole grains, fresh foods, raw or lightly steamed foods, fluids thrity minutes before or after meals (rather than with them), room temp beverages (if taken with meals), herb teas, fruit or vegetable juices, vegetable seasoning powder, kelp, goat's milk products, and foods that spoil.

We must listen to our bodies, too. If we take better care of our bodies now, it will take care of us later. As Dr. Jensen used to always say, "Take care of your body for the first fifty years, and it will take care of you for the next fifty years."

♥What about the nervous system?

If your body is stimulated on a physical level, with a chiropractic adjustment, let's say, it's also going to be stimulated on an emotional level by that adjustment as well. All of the emotions that go along with how your body ended up out of balance in the first place are going to be accessed and addressed.

> ♥Sometimes words are just inadequate. But the body speaks in volumes, energetically. ♥

Once an adjustment has been applied to the body, the energy centers within the body begin to flow and communicate along this massive network of electromagnetic cellular transmitters. The innate intelligence stimulates the pineal gland and hypothalamus (which is where all emotions are seated in the first place) and a higher vibration is able to permeate the lower vibrating tissues.

In other words, in an internal utter silence, energetically the healing begins.

There have been a great number of books written on the subject of vibration and energetic healing, the settling of emotion within the tissues and organs, and how the bodily discomfort we experience can be a direct message to us about how far out of alignment we are with our emotional selves.

Louis Hay, Carolyn Miss, and Chungliang Al Huang are all wonderful authors of such informative books on the subject of vibrational-emotional healing. I have added the names of their books in the library section found at the end of this chapter for your review.

Vibrational medicine is an absolutely fascinating field of study. I believe that each one of us has the ability to allow our hearts to speak its own language. When we do, we can become sensitive to the entire world in a completely different way than the way the brain sees the world.

Modern science is constantly learning more and more about energy fields and the fact that we are composed of more than just a physical structure. Science has even developed ways of measuring this energy, to some extent.

They use electrocardiograms (EKG) to measure currents from the heart and electroencephalograms (EEG) to measure electrical currents from the brain. They can measure the electro-potential of the skin with a lie detector machine, and magnetic fields around the body with a super-conducting quantum interference device that never even touches the body. They call it a SQUID machine and claim it can offer more information about the brain's functioning than a normal EEG can.

In 1959, Dr. Leonard Ravitz at William and Mary University showed that the Human Energy Field fluctuates with a person's mental and psychological stability, suggesting that there is a field associated with the thought processes.

There are massive changes in the way scientists are describing the physical body and physicists are now describing the physical universe. Scientists, physicists, and Spiritual healers are finding agreement on one aspect of the human structure: that there is a distinct energy of our hearts' "knowing" that is changing the way we interpret our self-definitions.

> ♥ The world of subjective human understanding is interconnecting to the scientific description of Newtonian physics and relativity theories. ♥

Okay, I know this may sound a little deep, but let me give you an example of what I am talking about. When I meet people with neck problems, let's say, there is generally a lot of self-imposed pressure associated with the individual's lifestyle. They generally have a feeling like the weight of the world is on their shoulders, and that they are responsible for taking care of everything.

There is a lot of service-oriented energy associated with the cervical spine. Sometimes I think people with neck pain find it easier to pretend they are pain-free, thus suppressing their emotions and their pain, simultaneously.

It's as if they believe that, if they were to turn their head through its full range of motion, it would in fact get all their body's information flowing and they would have to experience the feelings of the pressure and stress they are so busy running away from. So, for them it's just easier to live without turning their head…until the physical pain becomes more severe than the fears of the emotional pain they are suppressing.

Physically and emotionally our bodies vibrate. Crying is another form of healing and release. It's not necessarily a bad thing. Many people think it represents weakness, so we condition ourselves not to do it very often. But when crying comes after being suppressed for a long period of time, it's going to come big, with big, deep sobs. But again, this is all part of cleansing and letting it out.

As a natural healer, I'm telling you, I believe that the greatest weaknesses are not physical; they are emotional. Our bodies can find physical ways to express to us what's going on inside emotionally. Tears are just like over-flowing emotions. Journaling can really help with getting things up and out of the body. There is also a time and a place for counseling.

♥When Looking For a Healer♥

I find that most people go to therapy because they have a reason, but did you know that you don't have to have a *bad* life to know there is a *better* quality of life in store, if you seek out the appropriate information for your own healing.

There are really two schools of counseling—traditional clinical therapies and Christian, Laymen Faith counseling. The two can be in direct opposition to one another, at times. I believe self-help counseling works best when it is offered by those who share like Spiritual beliefs. You simply have more tools to draw on between the two of you.

When looking for a healer in any form, don't be afraid to ask about their personal beliefs. It is amazing how Spiritually void some healers can be. The fact is, if the healer is not dialed-in themselves, Spiritually speaking, who knows where their healing skills and inspirations are coming from?

> ♥ Your belief system is your foundation; it's your understanding of the un-anticipatable. It's your inner-communication and belief about yourself, life, and death. ♥

Now, those more skilled than you in the technicalities of articulatable beliefs and logical, rational thinking may be the people you want to seek out for advice, but don't ever let a counselor or healer tell you that faith is simply a crutch and serves no other purpose.

♥I think Faith may very well be the single most important part of your emotional psyche, and may be the very thing that keeps you alive when you have run out of words! ♥

History has demonstrated that the most notable winners usually encountered heartbreaking obstacles before they triumphed. They won because they refused to become discouraged by their defeats.

B.C. Forbes

♥ Constitutions:

Have you ever met anyone who can smoke, drink and party all night long, and it seems that they never get sick? Then you meet some people who have to wear a sweater when the slightest breeze blows, and they get sniffle anyway.

Well, this is what we call a strong or weak constitution. You don't get to choose which you will be born with, but you do get to choose what you're going to do with it. If you're feeling like, "my gosh, I'm taking vitamins, I'm doing all this work on myself and I'm still feeling worse then my smokin-drinkin-trashfood-eatin' friends," take heart. It may just be you're a weaker constitution. We cannot compare ourselves to anyone else when it comes to healing. Our structure is unique unto only us. We can look at it, analyze it, poke it, and prod it 'til the cows come home, but ultimately, you were born with certain strengths and weaknesses, and nature has seen fit to compensate us on both accounts.

The stronger structures may enjoy less focused attention to caring for their health needs; however, they will tend to be more analytical in life. The world will also expect them to carry the weight of the weaker structure's issues. These stronger structures may find themselves constantly sought after for advice or help from friends. The boss will look to them for overtime projects and families rely on those logical and linear thoughts during a crisis.

Stronger structures tend to suppress their emotions, fearing a softer side might weaken their resolve in some way. In a role assigned by society, admitting to being emotional, for a strong man, may appear to be unmasculine, so the expressive voice becomes the courage of the man (or woman).

When the expressive voice speaks from emotion derived in the head, rather than the heart, I find the words are less than compassionate, if you know what I mean. Focused time for relaxation and peace are a must for the constitutionally strong.

Those born with weaker constitutional structures are blessed with emotional access. What they lack in physical strengths, they make up for in sensitivity, compassion, and understanding. It's quite interesting that I have seen many a weaker constitution live a longer healthier, more balanced life-style than a stronger constitution, simply because they have learned to listen to their body's voice and work *with* their energy levels, rather than take advantage of them.

Having a strong or weak constitution is no guarantee that you will live a long and healthy life. Strong constitutions break down too, and when they do, they generally break in a big way. Weaker constitutions are reminded daily to care for themselves.

Weaker constitutions are the creators and carolers of this life. They paint the world the color of their hurts and their joys. If it's good, it's really good; if it's not, it's really not. Weaker structures need to be gentle to themselves and those around them. They wound deep over rejection and can be quite judgmental themselves.

Look for projects that inspire and lift the Spirits of those around you. Communication is very import, and again, journaling can help you stay in touch with what's going on inside of you.

Some experts have devoted their entire lives to reading the body. Scientists have spent millions of dollars trying to understand the chemistry of it. But what it all boils down to are some very basic rules.

> ♥ Do the best you can with what you were born with; don't try to be like anyone else, and listen to your body when it talks to you…it knows what you need, from the inside out. ♥

Of course, our bodies do have some basic chemical needs. But if you think you can meet all of those needs just by taking supplements, I would caution you. Most of our bodies' needs are met by eating, breaking down the foods we eat, and then absorbing specific parts of those foods (nutrients) into our system. I, as well as other natural health advocates, believe it's important to try to eat foods in a state that is as close to the way they are found in nature.

Why? Because Nature knows what she is doing when she grows a particular food. The plants seem to know just what nutrients to absorb from the ground, when to sprout a seed, and just what climate it will best grow in. When we eat these foods the way Nature grew them we get all the benefits of thousands of years of that innate intelligence.

If you think about it, man's wisdom is only as smart as our thoughts are at the time we think them, and we are constantly changing our minds. Man can take a carrot, cut it up, mix it with other things, and package it for easy microwaving. However, man has not yet figured out how to create the carrot in the first place.

All of the foods man has been able to create are devoid of life. We really don't know much about the long-term effects those foods that we have been able to genetically alter will have on our bodies. Are we poisoning ourselves with chemicals, preservatives, and additives? Only time will tell.

I am of the opinion that to keep the body in a balanced state, we should make an effort to eat a well-balanced diet, keeping the foods as close to the state it was grown in as possible. From there, we can move into convenience foods, supporting those choices with juicing and herbal supplementation.

I like to supplement with herbs because they are whole foods and plants. I find that most natural healing comes about when you add balance to the diet while supplementing with a whole food or herbal remedies, and working with the emotional and mental states, as well. That's not to say that I don't like vitamins, but vitamins are only components of foods, and they need foods to work with in the body, so my first choice will always be an herbal remedy.

Now, sometimes healing can be as simple as offering the body a few herbs with a meal and letting Nature and balance take its course, but that is the exception. There are some nutrients that, if taken alone, can actually be more damaging to the body than if they were taken in an herbal, or whole food state.

Let me give you an example. If you were to take a look at a good calcium supplement, hopefully you will find that it has been combined with magnesium and vitamin D.

Why? Because calcium can't be efficiently utilized by the body without magnesium and vitamin D to aid the process. Now, Nature already knows this, so when you are eating foods like kale, turnip greens, beet tops, cabbage, romaine lettuce, alfalfa sprouts, agar, almonds, avocados, coconut, kelp, goat's milk, and sesame seeds, you're getting some great calcium, and Nature has surrounded these foods, naturally, with all the other elements necessary for the body to recognize the calcium, provided that the body can break down the food.

If a person were to get his or her calcium out of the foods they ate, over the course of their lifetime, these foods would require the stimulation, digestion, elimination, absorption, and alkalization of the body as a whole.

Major deficiencies in certain nutrients, certainly, can result in serious disease, and even minimal deficiencies, over a long period, can affect our health. That is why supplementation is helpful, but, a well-balanced diet, open channels of elimination, and good digestion all play an import part in the overall picture of health.

Now, let's say that, over the course of a lifetime, someone who ate a good diet most of their life were to suffer from "thin bones," for instance. Deciding to take a calcium supplement without magnesium and vitamin D is not going to do much good. There are probably other factors involved in their overall picture; rather than just taking a supplement, they should look to find the reason the body is reacting the way it is to their lifestyle.

Calcium is one of the hardest things to digest and absorb, so this person may need to look at taking a digestive aid in order to break down the calcium from their foods. Poor digestion over the course of this person's lifetime could even be the heart of the problem in the first place, and certainly would be an area I would want to consider when taking any kind of remedy for "thin bones."

Are you starting to see the picture I am painting here? Again, this is an over-simplification to a potentially life-threatening condition, but my point is simply this: the body always responds perfectly to whatever situation in which it's been placed.

I am suggesting that we are never too old to begin a healthy eating regimen. A program of juice therapy, herbal supplementation, and a well-balanced diet is the best way to let Nature give you a helping hand.

♥ If you have a weakness, don't just take a supplement. Find out why your body is not absorbing those nutrients from the foods you're eating in the first place. And if you know you're not eating a balanced diet, that may be the first place to begin your work! ♥

♥What does the body need?

That being said, let's look at some of the body's needs from a chemical and nutritional perspective.

The adrenals and prostate need zinc. They can become depleted by over-consumption of refined carbohydrates in the typical "junk foods." As you eliminate processed foods and caffeine, and substitute fresh fruits and diluted, unsweetened fruit juices, you'll see your energy rise! The adrenals control metabolism of fats, carbohydrates, and proteins and help the pancreas regulate blood sugar levels. They watch over water and mineral balance, too, so you will want to avoid caffeine and aspirin, or anything that can over-stimulate the adrenals.

Protein is so important. Protein slows the digestion of carbohydrates, thereby reducing the strain on the adrenals. The brain is totally dependent upon blood sugar, and any fluctuations in its level can cause symptoms such as mood swings, depression, fatigue, cravings for sweets, weight problems, headaches, inability to concentrate, and/or a lack of energy. (Any of this sound familiar to you?)

The bones need fluorine, calcium, and phosphorus. Calcium helps to soothe the nerves, regulate blood cholesterol levels, control muscle function, build strong bones and teeth, offset cramping anywhere in the body, and assist in healing.

Get rid of the refined sugar and phosphorus-rich foods like luncheon meats and hot dogs. You might even want to limit red meats, too, because they rob the system of calcium. And don't be fooled by the TV commercials asking you if you have had your pasteurized or sweetened dairy products today. They provide little *usable* calcium to the body! Hydrochloric acid is important, because your body needs that to break down and aid in the absorption of calcium from foods and supplements.

We were talking about digestion earlier, but let's look a little closer at this very important body of energy. The digestive system needs chlorine, sodium and potassium. The nutrients we need to get out of our foods and supplements are only available to the cells if they are properly digested and absorbed.

We have to make sure that this system is working at its best. I think it's very important to support your digestive system whenever you're working with the other areas of the body. Heavy mucous in the body, allergies, a lack of energy, arthritis, gas, and bad breath can all be due to poor digestion.

Enzymes are necessary for the digestion of proteins, fats, and carbohydrates—in other words, all foods. Papaya and parsley can help encourage the stomach and liver to secrete its enzymes for digestion.

My Grandma would eat the aloe vera plant from her garden after a meal. She said it helped with digestion by providing a natural sodium balance for her stomach. Ginger, marjoram, tarragon, and rosemary all work well to help the body digest the toxic waste. I know what you're thinking—just eat a salad!

♥ Other Needs

Let's see, our hair needs silicon, the heart needs potassium (goat whey is a good source), the colon needs magnesium, the brain needs phosphorus, manganese, and sulfur. Vitamin C and peppermint can bring more oxygen to the brain. Gotu kola, capsicum, and Siberian ginseng have been traditionally used to feed the brain, as well.

The circulatory system needs sulfur, silicon, and oxygen. You have to watch the table salt and sea salt, as well as artificial sweeteners. Natural salts will not cause sodium imbalances in the system, so go for the vegetable seasoning broths and your circulatory system will love you for it!

The kidneys need chlorine and the lungs need oxygen; the liver needs sulfur and iron. The nervous system needs phosphorus, manganese and sulfur. The pituitary gland needs bromine, the skin needs sulfur, silicon, and oxygen, and the spleen needs fluorine and copper. The stomach needs chlorine and sodium, the teeth need fluorine, calcium, and phosphorus, the thyroid needs iodine, and our tissues need potassium, chlorine, and sulfur. Wow, what a mouthful!

♥ Minerals & Stuff

Our bodies also need inorganic substances such as calcium, iron, and magnesium, which are essential for the body to function. They are better known as minerals and act kind of like the spark plugs to the system. They don't do much by themselves, but they make the entire car run. Minerals do things like work with the chemical messengers in the body and the immune system, as well as build and repair body tissues.

There are other things, like amino acids and enzymes, too. Amino acids are a class of organic compounds found in foods, from which the building blocks of protein are constructed. There are at least twenty amino acids, eight of which cannot be manufactured in the body and must be obtained from our diet.

Then there are the enzymes, or proteins, that come from living cells and produce chemical changes by catalytic action (like digestion). Enzymes help break down food so nutrients can be utilized by the body, and are necessary for lots of other chemical processes that occur in the body, too.

Keeping all that in mind, you might be asking yourself right now, *How in the heck are we supposed to get all that stuff into our bodies?*

Well, since Nature put all this stuff in our foods for us, we just need to listen to her! She concentrates the necessary ingredients during different times of the year.

We need a full variety of foods to get all this stuff. Look at your diet. What do you think your cells are being made up of, just from today's meals? Personally, I think Nature kind of knows what she is doing. She has a formula and food for every one of her seasons.

Now, yes, there is truth to the claim that we are over polluting our waters, and dematerializing our soils, so that even naturally grown foods are becoming minerally devoid. Yet, somehow, Nature has still managed to find her way. Supplementing might be a good idea, and we talked about herbs.

♥ Herbs

Herbs are a good source of nutrients, because they are whole foods, capable of nourishing and supporting our body systems as a food. But there are also other things found in foods, such as fiber, and flavor, and they are essential to our health. We don't always call these things nutrients, even though lack of fiber and flavor can lead to poor immunity, fatigue, and other symptoms of decreased heath and even disease.

> ♥ Most healthcare concerns can be dealt with, optimistically, by proper nutrition, exercise, repletion, rest, and Spiritual peace. ♥

We don't necessarily have conscious control over how nutrients act in our bodies, but we do consciously choose the foods from which we are going to get them. Our government's daily nutritional recommendations suggest only nutrients that have been discovered by researchers.

There is a pretty good chance that there are others nutrients you are getting from your foods that science has not discovered, but that Nature knows we need. So, eating foods as close to Nature as possible—such as whole wheat, brown rice, and fresh fruits and vegetables—helps ensure that the body is getting ALL the nutrients it needs, known and unknown, in the way Nature intended.

Basically there are just a few things to keep in mind when healing with Nature:

1. Your foods should be whole, pure, and natural, in the proper proportions of 80% alkaline with 20% acid.
2. Your food must be taken in sufficient variety to meet the needs of every organ, gland, and tissue in the body and at least 60% raw (you need the live enzymes). Nature cures, but she must have the opportunity and the tools.
3. You must get enough sleep, and Nature will do the best she can with what she has to work with.

♥ How Fragile ♥

I am constantly amazed by how resilient the body was created to be, yet how fragile it can become when held up to our own free will. I find it hard to justify a diagnostic life-sentence for anyone willing to go through the natural phases of healing, therefore, I am constantly searching for Nature's healing truths.

So when it comes to natural healing, I believe that the mind can scream false information into our conscious realties, and our bodies are happy to interpret that information into physical reflection. I believe our greatest blunder in physical healing is the inconsistency with which we allow the Spirit to filter out the lies of our mind before the body grabs hold of those lies and makes them truths in the form of a physical disease.

> ♥I have found that, for every physical lesson my body has offered me, I've grown Spiritually, three times in proportion, if I've been open to the lesson of the illness. ♥

Learning to listen to what your body is trying to tell you can develop into a whole new way of communicating with truth.

Self♥Loving
the
Outside, Too:

In this section, you will find recipes for aroma therapies, Self♥Love potions, and lotions that I think complete the entire picture of Self♥Loving ♥moments, spent alone with you.

♥Body Lotion Potions!

Well-brushed skin, smeared with a warmly scented or fabulously fragrant Self♥Love body lotion, can be a persuasive way to catch someone's attention, or just make you feel great all over. Most of these potions you can prepare right in your very own kitchen, because they are largely made of water and oil. Nearly all of my lotions, sprays, and scrub recipes are highly nutritive, moisturizing, and emollient.

Let's talk about the three main ingredients required to make a lotion or cream. First, there is the "liquid" oil portion of the lotions. I love olive oil with lavender and rose petals, soaked for eight weeks. The heavier the oils you use, the oilier the lotion will be going onto your skin. Once you get the hang of lotion making, you will find many different oils, mixes, and other options from which to choose. There are oils such as peanut, jojoba, apricot, macadamia nut, sweet almond, wheat germ, sesame oil, and so on, however, I find the peanut and sesame oils to be a little too nutty smelling for my preference. For a lighter feel, I like to use fractionated coconut oils. Once you have made a batch or two, you'll learn what oils work best for you. Experiment until you find just the right recipe for you.

Second, there is the "solid oil" portion of your lotion. When I say solid, I'm talking about those oils that are solid at room temperature, like coconut oil-76, cocoa, mango, shea butters, and even some powders. But the key is, when these oils are heated, they melt to a pour. When they sit a room temperature, they become solid again. This is what helps make the lotions and creams thick.

And, third, there is the "water portion." The water portion can be made from distilled waters, floral waters, witch hazel, herbal infusions, aloe gel, herbal tinctures, glycerin, and other water-soluble ingredients. The more water you use, the more liquid a cream you will get.

I love to use aloe and glycerin. Glycerin adds a nice soothing and healing property to the lotions. I like to add natural preservatives, as well, such as grapefruit seed extract or vitamins A, C, or E. Some essential oils are great natural preservatives, too. When I use essential oils in lotions, I use about 2½ to 3 teaspoons of essential oil per 20 oz of lotion, but you can use more or less, depending on your preference.

My favorite lotion recipe requires a mix of 6 to 7 oz liquid oil, 2 to 3 oz solid oil, 1 oz beeswax, 9 oz distilled water and 10 to 40 drops of your favorite fragrant or medicinal essential oil. This recipe will give you anywhere from 16 to 20 oz of luscious, creamy lotion. For a thick and rich cream, the inner phase should be about one-half of the outer phase with the emulsifying agent, comprising no more than 5 to 20 % of the oil.

> ♥I know that sounds really technical, but it's all quite simple, once you get started. ♥

♥A basic Self♥Love Potion Lotion

Before you begin, you should become familiar with the **"Safe Ingredient Handling Tips"** in the back of this section. After you have become familiar with the safety requirements, assemble all of your ingredients on your workstation.

You will need:

> 6 oz of "liquid oil"
> 16 oz heatproof measuring cup
> 3 oz solid oil
> 1 oz beeswax
> a pot, partially filled with water
> a medium heat potholder
> a spoon or stir stick
> a blender
> very clean, dry jars with lids

Start by sterilizing your bottles, jars, and equipment before use. A dishwasher works just fine. I find that one part bleach to four parts water, used as a rinse, works nicely, too. Don't use wooden utensils, as they can harbor bacteria that can overwhelm your lotions natural preservatives.

Pour 6 oz of your selected liquid oil into a 16 oz heatproof measuring cup. If you are using herb infused oils, you must strain the oils from the herbs in the bottle. Now, place the cup into a pot partially filled with water and give it a medium heat.

Keep the temperature between 100 and 160 degrees to avoid damaging the oil properties. A candy thermometer works just fine.

Next, add your pre-selected 3 oz of solid oil to the liquid oil in the cup. If you haven't pre-measured it, you can simply add the solid oil pieces to the oil until the total volume reaches the 9 oz mark on the measuring cup. This will give you an exact 3 oz measurement.

Add 1 oz or so of the beeswax to the cup in the same way. You should have a total volume of about 10 oz. You may want to add more or less after you have experimented with your first batch.

Stir the mixture until the oils and beeswax melt and dissolve into the liquid. Then, remove the cup from the hot water and allow the oils to cool until it's comfortable to touch the cup to your wrist. As it cools, the mixture will become thick, so, you must stir it once or twice to keep the consistency smooth and uniform. If it becomes cooler than body temperature, just reheat.

While the oils are cooling, pour 8 to 9 oz of distilled water into a clean measuring cup and heat to body temperature. You can place it into the hot-water bath after the oil mixture has been removed from the heat, or blend the water on high in the Vita-mixer, until it is warmed slightly.

Test the temperature of your water, and, when the oil mixture and the water have both reached about the same temperature, you're ready to begin the whipping portion of your potions.

If you are going to add a preservative, you will want to do so at this point. Preservatives are used to defeat bacteria, yeast, and fungi growth that consume the fixed oils in lotions. Since microorganisms can only grow in water, the active form of the preservative must be added in the water phase for it to be effective. I like to use vitamin C, or grapefruit seed extract. I also like to add a little Polysorbate 20 in the water phase to help disperse and emulsify the oils.

Pour the warmed water (strained, if you are using an herb infused water) into a clean blender or food processor, along with any added water-soluble ingredients. Process at high speed in a regular blender or the low speed on a Vita-mixer.

Now comes the most fun, and most important part, of lotion making—the processing. This is where the inner (oil) phase should be slowly added to the outer (water) phase. Slowly trickle the oil mixture to the whirling water. As you add a thin downpour into the spiraling water, you will see the lotion begin to thicken. This happens rather quickly.

Continue to process until the oil and water have blended together into a thick, creamy liquid. About 5 to 10 minutes in a blender and about 30 seconds in a Vita-mixer. When the water and oil combine into one liquid, you have a cream.

Once the cream begins to thicken in the blender, quickly begin to pour the cream into your clean, dry jars, filling them to the top and leaving as little airspace as possible. Your mixture will thicken as it cools, so work quickly. You may now add more essential oils, if you like, and stir them right into the jar. Place the tight-fitting, self-sealing lids on the jars, and date and label them.

Store the cream out of direct heat and sunlight. Depending on the ingredients, they won't last much past a month or so. You can refrigerate them for longer storage, but unfortunately, cold temperatures can change the consistency of a cream. The water might bead out and the solid oils may turn granular. It does not change the effectiveness of the cream, but might not look so great if you are giving it as a gift. If the cream should separate after a period of time, whip it back up again and drop a little pinch of borax into the mix, while slightly warming the cream, to re-emulsify it.

Organic natural creams are hard to come by, because they are so perishable, but, no doubt, they are worth the effort. Have fun with your Lotions & Potions, but, use them up quickly, then make some more! Depending on the essential oils you add to your lotions, you can get a different experience with each jar. Next, I want to show you how to make a salve.

♥Grandmas Healing Salves

It was my grandma that taught me to keep my pantry good and stocked with herbs and spices, just in case of emergencies. She was always pulling something or other out of her kitchen cabinets, for everything from my daughter's skinned knees to grandpa's chapped hands, and my own sunburns and chapped lips. It was always fun to see just what she was going to whip up next. She had a fix for just about anything.

By stocking your cabinets with a few extra ingredients, you too can make the following simple recipes when you're caught in a pinch. They work great for everyday troubles too!

Olive oil is my preferred choice of oil when I am making a salve, because the skin just loves olive oil, and accepts it easily. I'll add herbs, like dried comfrey, calendula, burdock root, and lavender to the olive oil portion of the salve.

Keep in mind, olive oil is heavy and carries a strong odor of its own. If I find myself in need of an ointment, and don't have any herb infused olive oils in my pantry, I'll just use olive oil by itself in the salve, and just add a couple of extra drops of essential oils to the jar before I put the lid on it.

Although essential oils and herb infused oils are not interchangeable, and have different healing properties to them, you can still get a good healing salve with either method. If the salves or oils start to smell aged, it's time to use it to polish your shoes and furniture, and make some new batches.

If your sniffer can't tell the difference, run a little basil under your nose and then smell the salve again. Grammy used to tell me that basil will balance out your sense of smell. Wonder if that's why she used so much of it in her cooking.

♥ Making a Salve

1½ oz olive oil
½ oz beeswax
¼ teaspoon healing essential oil

Once I make a salve, I store it in ¼ to ½ oz tin or plastic containers. I'll give my neighbors and friends the extras, because each batch will make more than I can use before they go bad, unless I am sunburnt from head to toe.

Warm the olive oil in a heatproof measuring glass, by placing the cup in a pot filled half way with water. Add the beeswax and continue to warm until the wax melts.

If you want to test your salve consistency, dip a very clean frozen metal spoon into the oils then touch the cooled oil on the spoon with your finger. If you decide you want a harder salve (like in the Summertime), just add more beeswax to the oil. This is how you make lip balms, too. Make them a little on the harder side (2 oz oil to 1 oz beeswax)—that way they won't seep out of the jar and into your makeup drawer or purse on a hot Summer day!

Once you have the consistency you want, remove the cup from heat and cool only slightly. It will begin to thicken quickly, so have your jars, tins, or tubes ready. Pour the salve into the containers and let them cool. They will get harder as they cool.

If you are going to add essential oils to the salve, do it before they cool completely. Then, put the tops on the bottles and jars to keep the volatile essential oils from evaporating.

I use anywhere from 8-15 drops of essential oil per ¼ tin. By adding the essential oil of Wintergreen or birch to the salve, you end up with a great analgesic for painful or swollen joints. If you add tea tree oil, rosemary, and lavender, you get a terrific antiseptic for dry, broken skin.

If you want to make a rich, thick balm instead of a salve, just adjust the recipe to 1 oz cocoa or mango butter, plus 1 oz olive oil, 1 oz jojoba oil, 2 oz shea butter (which has a very strong smell) and 1 oz beeswax.

Melt this all down in the same way and pour into a jar (one big enough to get your hand into). Add your oils and smear some over your dry chapped hands and feet before you go to bed. Pull a pair of warm and cozy socks over your hands and feet, and you will love your skin come morning time!

♥Essential Oils and Aromatherapy♥

Aromatherapy is the ancient art of using essential oils for promoting health and well-being. Essential oils are the vital life essences, extracted from certain aromatic plants and flowers.

For centuries, and all throughout the Bible, we see references to the resins from the frankincense tree, myrrh, aloes, cassia, cedarwood, cypress, spikenard, hyssops, and so on, to be used for healing, strengthening, purifying, and cleansing.

There is a clear pattern for the cleansing and purifying use of oils in the Old Testament of the Bible in Exodus 30:22-25. The Lord gave Moses a very specific recipe to be used for an "oil of holy ointment," explaining, down to the last detail, which oils and herbs were to be combined, and in what measures to make this powerful, natural healing substance.

Our sense of smell is the only one of the five senses directly linked to the limbic lobe and the thalamus of the brain. Anxiety, depression, fear, anger, as well as joy, peace, and all positive emotions emanate from this region, so the effect of essential oils can have a profound healing effect on both body and mind.

The use and application of specific oils, along various parts of the body, or simply diffused into the air around us, may help us to make leaps and bounds full of progress in our health care and Self♥Loving routines.

Research has only just begun to delve into the realm of the subconscious mind, and how emotions affect every aspect of our lives and bodies. Most people consider periods of great confusion, uncertainty, depression, or insecurity to be a normal part of modern day living, but that's not the way we were designed to live! There are a lot of people unable to progress forward in real life issues, or unable to achieve their goals and dreams, even with traditional forms of psychological therapy, because past emotional patterns are locked so deep within the DNA that they have a hard time just getting to the issues.

According to Dr. Gary Young, we carry in our cells the programming of our ancestors for four generations, and new knowledge is coming forth, everyday, as research continues.

> ♥ Synthetic chemicals can generally only do one thing at a time. Essential oils, however, can perform several functions at the same time, giving them a paradoxical nature that can be difficult to understand. ♥

If you think about it, we human beings are paradoxical in nature, as well. You know, a mom can be a wife, friend, co-worker, church volunteer, etc. And so the same might be said of the benefits of using essential oils. One oil can have several different uses, yet remain the same oil. An individual oil may have as many as 800 different chemical constituents, with only 200 of them having been "officially identified" and grouped into hydrocarbons and oxygenated compounds by science.

♥ Applications:

The feet, ears, and wrists are areas of the body that can absorb oils the fastest, because of the large pores. Vita Flex Therapy (which is a simple method of applying oils to contact points or nerve endings in the feet or hands) is also a great way to apply oils to specific body points. Generally, 6-10 drops of an oil is sufficient. (Again, read the safety handling instructions and get professional advice before applying any oil to your body).

Dilute your essential oils 10-35% in what's called a carrier oil, if you are going to massage a larger area of the body, or large muscles. Carrier oils are oils like olive, macadamia nut, or even the Self♥Love potions and lotions we just learned how to make! Always dilute your essential oils before applying to small children.

If you take a bath, you can add oils to the water, or shower gel base, and take a nice long soak. If you massage an area after a hot shower, the pores of the body will be open, and the oils will be accepted deeper into the tissues.

You can diffuse the oils into the air with an aromatic diffuser. Place 10-25 drops of undiluted essential oil in a nebulizing diffuser. Some use light bulbs, others hot water. Even forced-air fans will help circulating the oils and disperse them into the air, oxygenating and improving the quality of the air.

You can even smell them right out of the bottle. You can put one or two drops of oil on a tissue cotton ball, pillow case etc., and just inhale it, or slip the cotton ball into your bra for the wonderful fragrance all day. There are so many ways to use fragrance! Learn to trust your nose. The library and the Internet are great sources of information.

♥ Raindrop Therapy:

This particular term was coined by Dr. Don Gary Young, N.D., one of North America's leading experts on the art and science of aromatherapy.

The "Raindrop" technique involves dropping oils directly onto the spine and working them into the body by using light massage strokes, which stimulates energy impulses and disperses the oils along the nervous system, throughout the entire body. The oils will continue to work in the body anywhere from one to four weeks.

It is thought to bring about balance and energy to the vital centers of the body. Dr. Young suggests that applications done in this way may even *"kill viruses that hibernate along the spinal column."*

I have adapted Dr. Young's technique with my own personal additions, which enhance the treatments further. A basic raindrop treatment will generally include the use of rosewood, blue tansy, frankincense, and spruce, which may help balance the electrical energies within the body and create an environment where structural alignment can occur. I love to use this combination on the bottom of my feet and along my spine after a chiropractic adjustment, as well.

Dr. Young suggests thyme, oregano, cypress, birch, basil, pepermint, marjoram, and, finally, a combination essential and mixing oil that will relax the major muscles of the body.

I like to specifically test my clients for the substitute oils their body may be calling for (using muscle-testing and various other sensitivity indicators), and I will apply assorted single or combination oils along the body's energy fields. As an acupuncturist might use needles to move energy, I use oils and touch, instead.

The object is to develop a new memory in the tissues of the body and train the body to accept and hold that new memory. Many times we will get emotional clearing from years past, in one single session!

♥A Visit

After returning from a visit with a wonderful healer friend of mine who lives in Canada, I received a call asking about the raindrop session I had given her while I was there. Mind you, she is on the threshold of recognizing her own healing talents, and is contemplating her ability to share her gifts with others. My visit to her home was to help her see her gifts, as well as facilitate the path in which she would share them with the world.

Here is an excerpt of a letter I wrote to her responding to her questions regarding the influence of essential oil therapy and emotions. Although you are not privy to all of the circumstances that took place before the writing of this letter, my purpose in sharing this information with you is to offer you encouragement in your own Self♥Loving path, and to demonstrate the wide range of influence essential oils can have.

> …Crying is okay, and yes, a desire to move closer to Spirit is common. The body does not know how to hurt; it only knows how to heal! Trust yourself—you will be led; just keep praying for the truth. You can't learn it ALL in one day, darlin! Give yourself some time. As a healer, you will be tested by the world, but because you are a healer, you don't want to identify with the pain. You have to listen for what it is the body wants to change. Where you are the most protective in your life is where you are also the most ignorant. I don't mean that in a nasty way. I simply mean, if you are feeling frustrated, you are not educating yourself and your body with the information it's hungry for (and, after raindrop, perhaps more open to). On some level, fear, danger, even crisis moves us to change. Perhaps this is the way your DNA is moving you into that change. Are you journaling? Are you seeking Spiritual enlightenment? By now, the immediate effects of the raindrop will have worn off, and the old patterns are returning to the structure. But, know this: as healers we don't FIX cells (or problems). I cannot improve on that which is perfect; I can only help your body slough off the old and imperfect and make room for the new. If you are identifying with sadness, negativity and the fear of moving forward into your role as a natural healer (which has probably been heightened, following your raindrop) you do not have in place a way of nourishing the positive, uplifting, enlightening side of your life, so STOP what

you are doing! You are just more aware of what already exists in your life, after a raindrop. Healing takes time and a willingness to look at your toxins as they pass from you. If you don't do that, then you're not going to heal, and you're just going to feel the effects of toxins brought to the surface of your life. Get what I'm saying? God's abundance is available to everyone! You're a great healer. Claim it, and trust it's not coming from you, but through you. Now, yes, you do need to clear yourself, because you don't want to take on the negative emotions that are being released from those that you are working with, and we will talk more about how to do this, later. This may be part of your frustration right now, but don't doubt yourself. If you do, this higher vibration is slowly prohibited from flowing (old patterns return), and the body mourns for that higher vibration. When your progress stops, it's usually because you have run out of gratitude. Each challenge brings its own rewards, so, contribute to your own happiness by allowing your body to heal through daily documentation, proper nutrition, Spiritual enlightenment, peaceful surroundings, and appropriate education, then you will stop interfering with God's regeneration process, and healing will occur—not only in your body, but in your practice, as well. It flows all around you, through you, and to others! If your Spiritual doors are open to conflicting energy, you're going to feel the struggle for your peace of mind IN your mind. Healing comes from God, from the top down, inside out. Even subtle energy has an effective force! I would suggest you take those necklaces off and reevaluate their use in your life. Take a salt bath or shower, pray for each person on your healing list, in God's name, each day for seven days. Read inspiring Spiritual literature during those 7 days. Eat only LIVE foods. At the end of the seven days, your journaling will reveal the source of your unhappiness or frustration.

Remember, you are particles and waves—cells, multiplying and transforming information. It's all demonstrating the higher power, the life force of God. Don't stop the process. Okay, so, I hope that answers your question. I'm not even going to re-read what I just wrote you. Felt like I was on a roll there. I hope I didn't say anything that offends.

Love ya
Mwahhhh!

When I am performing a raindrop, I like to stimulate as many of the senses of the body (with the exception of taste) as possible. I play music (with guided imagery and positive affirmations), the rooms are visually peaceful—the body is warmly stimulated and lovingly nurtured as the wonderfully uplifting aromas come together to create a totally peaceful experience. I ask my raindrop clients to bring their own towels, and I will apply these oils onto those towels so after their showers throughout the week they will be reminded of their peaceful experience.

> ♥ Because of the effect of scents on the limbic lobe of the brain, essential oils can be profoundly healing to both mind and body. ♥

I will send each client home (in some cases with a specialized refer-ral), along with reading, journaling, and nutrition homework, bath salts, body oils, or color therapy. I've worked along side a myriad of psy-chologists, marriage and family counselors, chiropractors, and, yes, even medical doctors, who find their patients are just not progressing as rapidly as they would like. Negative emotions can be brought forward in your DNA, from up to four generations back, and the use of scents, touch, and sound can open passages to healing when other therapies have been unsuccessful.

If you are going to try this on yourself, you will have to use an application called Vita Flex Therapy (which involves applying oils to the bottoms of the feet). Be sure you read up on the side effects of each oil you choose to use. The best raindrop therapies I have ever experienced have come from those healers with whom I share like Spiritual beliefs, and who are Spiritually grounded as well as cultured in energy work.

♥Sometimes the best healers can be your very own grandmas! ♥

♥Oils, My Personal Favorites

Here is a list of some of my personal favorite oils and their traditional uses, however, please keep in mind that this information is not intended to diagnose, prescribe, or treat any disease, illness, or injured condition of the body. Please consult your local natural health care professional for more information.

Basil is relaxing to spastic muscles and is stimulating to the nerves and the adrenal cortex.

Bergamot has uplifting and stimulating properties to it that support the body in conditions of fatigue, stress, or depression. The oral herbal supplement, St. John's Wort has gained worldwide recognition for its ability to alleviate mild to moderate depression, without unpleasant side effects. (Never combine St. John's Wort with other prescription medications for depression.) I like to blend bergamot with lavender, mandarin, Roman chamomile, and Bulgarian rose when I am working with comforting negative emotions.

Birch is great for removing discomfort associated with the inflammation of bones, muscles, and joints. It may also help cleanse the lymphatic system.

Cinnamon is one oil you always want to use well diluted. The warming properties of cinnamon comfort and soothe the body and mind. It's peppery, sweet, and spicy. It's one of the best antivirals I know of, and I like to mix it with frankincense and mandarin. Careful, this one can really irritate the skin, so I use it with misters and diffusers more than topically.

Cypress is used for its antibacterial, antiinfectious, and diuretic properties. In addition, it may function as a decongestant for the circulatory and lymphatic systems.

Clary Sage helps balance and warm. This is a great oil for PMS and menopause. I like to massage it over the lower back and abdomen, and combine it with nutmeg, Bulgarian rose, geranium, and lavender to help balance out the female glandular system. Oral supplements of Dong Quai, red raspberry leaves, and some soy products are also very helpful when using these oils.

Eucalyptus stimulates the entire respiratory system and encourages movement. Put a little horse-radish under your tongue and rub some eucalyptus over your chest and "Whammo!" I also like to use boneset herb, fennel seeds, fenugreek, and mullein leaves as a tea or oral supplement, to help get things moving, and then combine the essential oils of geranium, peppermint, and rosemary with eucalyptus, and rub that on my back and chest to help support the respiratory system, as well.

Frankincense has been popular since ancient times. It's centering and comforting. Its antimicrobial and astringent properties make it useful for the skin, especially mature or dry skin. I like to mix it with bergamot, geranium, lavender, lemon, patchouli, pine needles, rosemary, and sandalwood. Works well with all the skin care products I've ever created

Geranium is one rosy, sweet, and flowery fragrance. It's balancing, calming and uplifting. It has antimicrobial properties and is widely used in skin care because of its ability to restore balance to oily and dry skin and hair. It's gentle enough for sensitive skin too. I love to mix it with lavender fine, and Bulgarian rose. Wonderful for the lymphatic system!

Jasmine is rich, warm, exotic, and sweet! Oh I love this oil for its history of use as an aphrodisiac. It has antispasmodic and antidepressive properties and is especially helpful for menstrual concerns and dry sensitive skin. Mix it with Bulgarian rose and WOW!

Lavender Fine has a mellow fragrance that balances and soothes the nervous system. It calms the body under stress and helps reduce tension and anxiety. It works great with oral B-complex supplementation. For emotional grounding under stress, I like to combine bergamot, geranium, neroli, Roman chamomile, and Bulgarian rose with fine lavender for a wonderfully restful sleep.

Lemon is bright, sharp, fresh, and stimulating. Works great on the abdomen and supports the body during over acidic conditions. I love to combine it with peppermint to stimulate digestion. It works great with herbal supplements of digestive enzymes that break down protein, carbohydrates, and fats.

Mandarin is mild, soft, and citrus fresh. Its cheerful aroma is invigorating and uplifting. It has wonderful astringent properties which work great for skin toning. It has natural antioxidants to help protect skin as well.

Marjoram is used to relax spastic muscles, soothe the nerves, relieve cramps, aches, and pains, and to help calm the respiratory system.

Oregano works in conjunction with thyme to strengthen the immune system, and to attack bacteria and viruses. It may also act as an antiseptic for the respiratory system, help balance metabolism, and strengthen the vital centers of the body.

Peppermint is used to calm and strengthen the nerves, reduce inflammation, and is highly effective when dealing with conditions related to the respiratory system, It also has a synergistic and enhancing effect on all other oils.

Pink Grapefruit is a warm, fresh, sweet oil, traditionally used for its toning and stimulating properties. It is astringent, antimicrobial, uplifting and soothing. It's great for oily skin and hair and works wonders on cellulite and fluid retention.

Pine Needle is a fresh, forest-like aroma that is stimulating uplifting and warming. It is so soothing to the skin and I love to use it in my detox recipes although you must be careful if you have kidney weakness or sensitive skin. The aroma helps with respiratory concerns and acts as a wonderful household deodorizer.

Rosemary is stimulating and warming while promoting circulation, and it acts like a tonic. It also works great on the feet and abdomen. I love to use it in my hair!

Roman Chamomile soothes and cools for hot, inflammatory conditions. The oral supplements of glucosamine, and chondroitin are useful in maintaining healthy joint and connective tissue. I like to blend Roman chamomile with clove bud, ginger, and nutmeg for a warming, penetrating soothing massage for joints.

Thyme is used for its ability to support the immune system, by attacking any bacteria, fungus infection or virus that may be present. It may also help one overcome fatigue and physical weakness after an illness.

♥ Healing Combinations:

Basil, Lavender, Cypress, and Marjoram may help to relax, calm, and relieve the tension of spastic muscles resulting from sports injury, fatigue, or stress.

Rosewood, Blue Tansy, Frankincense, and Spruce may help balance the electrical energies within the body and create an environment where structural alignment can occur. I love to use this combination on the bottoms of my feet and along my spine after a Chiropractic adjustment. It just makes me feel stronger.

Sandalwood, Juniper, Frankincense, Myrrh, Angelica, and Spruce may help to open the subconscious mind through pineal stimulation, to release deep-seated trauma encoded in the DNA, and bring a sense of grounding through elevated Spiritual consciousness. Put a couple of drops on the crown of the head. I find it helps me when I am struggling with accepting others with an open heart. In other words, it helps diminish my ego!

Hyssop, Spruce, Lavender, Sikenard, Geranium, Frankincense, Ylang Ylang, Orange, Sandalwood, Angelica, Sage, Bulgarian Rose, and Neroli is an exquisite harmonic fragrance which may promote physical and emotional healing, bringing about balance and allowing communication to flow more efficiently through the body. It may help reduce stress, and I find it creates a general overall feeling of well-being. I place a couple of drops directly on or along the side of the body.

Bulgarian Rose, Melissa, Helichrysum, Angelica, Frankincense, Sandalwood, and Lavender may help release negative memory and emotions, in order to forgive and forget, and get on with your life. Apply around navel or wear as a perfume.

Bulgarian Rose, Bergamot, Mandarin, Ylang Ylang, Lemon, and Geranium may help produce a magnetic energy to enhance the frequency of Self♥Love. I love this combination, as it brings back memories of being loved, being held, and sharing loving moments. When we have grief, the adenoids and the adrenal glands shut down, but the feelings of love (yes, even Self♥Love) and joy can open these centers right back up. Apply over the heart.

Neroli, Ylang Ylang, and Spruce may have an empowering effect which gives a feeling of being *"in the moment."* One can only go forward and progress when in the present time. Apply over the thymus.

Ylang Ylang, Lavender, Geranium, Sandalwood, and Blue Tansey may help release anger and frustration, bringing about a sense of peace and emotional well-being. I like to apply it over the liver area.

Orange and Tangerine may stimulate memory response and help you reconnect to your youthful side. One of the first steps to finding emotional balance is to connect with one's identity. When we become disconnected from our inner child or identity, it can cause confusion in our mid-adult years, often labeled as mid-life crisis. Apply around navel and nose.

Spruce and Sage may help ground us, in order to deal logically with reality, in a peaceful manner. When not grounded, it is easy to make choices which lead to bad relationships and bad business decisions. We escape because we don't have anchoring or awareness as to how to deal with the emotions. This combination may be helpful when we disconnect from reality, either because we are excited about new ideas, or want to escape into a protective fantasy. Apply to brain stem, back of neck, and sternum.

Melissa, Spruce, Juniper, Myrrh, Roman Chamomile, and Ylang Ylang may help you reconnect with a feeling of hope for tomorrow. It may also help with overcoming depression. Hopelessness can cause a loss of vision of growth and dreams. Massage on outer edge of the ears.

Lavender, Chamomile, and Orange Blossom is my signature blend. It's my personal Self♥Love potion fragrance. When one inhales the combination of these three oils, they are immediately able to relax. It is uplifting, refreshing and arousing! Apply over navel, chest, or diffuse.

♥Blending Your Own Combinations

If you are just beginning, do some homework, one oil at a time. Remember, you can always buy pre-mixed essential oils, which takes the guesswork out of it for you. You will learn to let your nose be your guide, while your brain accumulates the information about the medicinal properties of your blends. To blend oils, you need to know the break down of the oils, and the order in which they should be blended, in order to keep the therapeutic properties alive. I have listed some basic blending information below, but don't get confused. It's all really quite simple.

The Personifier is generally 1 to 5% of a blend, and has strong properties associated with its therapeutic actions.

The Enhancer is anywhere from 50 to 80% of a blend, and is the predominate oil. It's used to "enhance" the properties of the other oils used.

The Equalizer is 10 to 15% of a potion, and used to create a balance to the oil.

The Modifier is 5 to 8 % of a blend, and used to harmonize a blend.

When you are using strong essential oils, one drop can be very powerful. Some oils will also be thicker than others, so, 25 drops of one oil may make ¼ teaspoon, while it takes 30 drops of another to make the same measurement. Therefore, know your conversion tables when measuring drops, drams, milliliters and teaspoons.

Generally speaking:

25-30 drops = ¼ tsp

45-50 drops = ½ tsp

75-80 drops = ¾ tsp

100-120 drops = 1 tsp, and so on.

Follow your nose when creating, but check out some good books on the subject. When it comes to blending oils, you may want to know the constituents and chemical effects of each of the variables, so, I have listed a few here:

Sesquiterpenes: Antiseptic and anti-inflammatory, soothing, sedative.

Farenesene: Antiviral action

Limonene: Strong antiviral properties found in 90% of the citrus oils.

Pinene: Antiseptic and found in high proportions in the conifer oils such as pine and fir.

Esters: Compounds resulting from the reaction of an alcohol with an acid. They can be very relaxing and antifungal.

Aldehydes: Highly reactive and characterized by the group C-H-O (Carbon-Hydrogen, and Oxygen). Can be irritating to the skin and have a lemon like scent.

Ketones: Can be a neuro-toxin when isolated from other constituents. Dissolves mucous and fats.

Phenols: Responsible for the fragrance of an oil. Can be potentially irritating to the liver and stimulating to the nervous system.

Oxides: Radical oxygen. Expectorant.

My two favorite companies to order pre-mixed and single oils from are *Nature's Sunshine* and *Young Living*. They both have very high standards of testing and extracting oils. These oils may cost a little more, but they are worth it. So are you for that matter. You be your own judge. I have listed their numbers in the resource section of this book, so you can call the companies directly and order these oils at wholesale prices, even if you don't have a resale number.

Use caution and get professional advice before applying any oil to your body, especially if you are pregnant. Please read the safety handling tips located at the back of this section. Here are a few recipes you can use to make wonderful potions using only a handful of single essential oils and household items.

Effective & Effortless Recipes

A Lady's Washroom Secrets
Foundational Bath Salt
1/3 cup salts, such as Epsom salt, or fine or coarse sea salts.
7-12 drops essential oils

Mix your salts in glass bowls with wooden spoons. Try different combinations of essential oils, being sure to understand the precautions of each oil before you use them.

A Detoxifying Soak
This bath will help draw out body toxins, re-mineralize the body, and stimulate the lymphatic system.

2-3 thin slices of ginger	½ cup sea salts
2 tablespoons jojoba oil	1/8 cup glycerin
No more than 5 drops pink grapefruit	4 drops geranium
7 drops thyme	1 cup Moore mud or clay

Add the essential oils to the sea salts first and stir them in with a wooden spoon. Next, blend the jojoba into the salts and add the glycerin as well. Pour mixture into tub under warm running water and add the slices of ginger. Slip into the warm water and be sure to drink plenty of cool Spring water as you perspire.

Mineral Marinade for the Body.

½ cup fine dead sea salts	¼ cup borax (a natural mineral)
¼ cup baking soda	10 drops lavender
6 drops geranium	5 drops pink grapefruit
7 drops bergamot	

Enough for two baths. Mix essential oils in the sea salts first, then add the borax and baking soda. This recipe will soften and re-mineralize your skin. It's great for detox, too. Add some ginger and lemon slices, if you like, to the warm bath water, or to your cool drinking water. Smooth on some Self♥Love Potion lotions after your bath, or add one teaspoon of the following recipe to your soak water for an extra moisturizing bath.

Want a bath oil that disappears in your bath water? Try this lighter recipe:

½ cup massage oil   1/8 cup vegetable glycerin
1/8 cup castile soap   add your essential oils

After-Bath Moisturizing Oil

½ cup oil—massage oil, olive oil etc.   1 teaspoon jojoba oil
4 capsules of vitamin E, opened   2 drops geranium
7 drops sandalwood   4 drops lavender
1 drop peppermint

For more sensual fragrance, use 2 drops jasmine, ylang ylang, clove, and geranium, with 3 drops sandalwood, 1 drop patchouli and 5 drops bergamot. Place your ingredients in a glass bottle and mix it up. Rub it onto the skin after bathing and before toweling off. Do not expose your skin to direct sunlight following application.

Easy Natural Shower Gels

¼ cup castile soap   2 tablespoons aloe vera gel
1 teaspoon jojoba oil   1 capsule B complex (for color)
1 drop myrrh or frankincense
11 drops each of lavender, mandarin, and pink grapefruit

Combine all these ingredients in a measuring cup and pour into a plastic squeeze bottle. If you want to color the gel yellow, break open a B complex capsule or add a drop of red beet juice.

Naturally Fragrant Soaps

Use about 4 ounces of clear, solid glycerin to 20-25 drops of essential oils. All you need to do is melt the glycerin in a double boiler and add the essential oils. Pour into ice cube trays or soap molds and let cool.

Pop them out once cooled and there you have natural soaps. You can even add slices of ginger, lavender, peppermint leaves etc to spice the soaps up a little. Use your imagination and have fun! If you are giving them as gifts, attach a little note tag explaining what the essential oils you have chosen to use will do for them.

Great alternative combinations

1) 15 drops lavender, 5 drops peppermint
2) 6 drops lemon, 10 drops bergamot & grapefruit, 4 drops mandarin
3) 2 drops jasmine, 2 drops Bulgarian Rose, 3 drops ylang ylang

Bubble Baths

¼ cup chamomile tea or purified water   ½ teaspoon fine sea salt
1 cup castile soap   4 teaspoons vegetable glycerin
7 drops geranium   8 drops lemon
4 drops Roman Chamomile   3 drops lavender
2 drops Jasmine (if you have it some or Bulgarian Rose and Ylang Ylang)

Mix salt and tea or water together. Then, add castile soap and mix in the glycerin and essential oils, and stir it up. Transfer the mixture into a beautiful glass bottle that pours easily. This will give you about 2 baths and should be used within 3-5 days. For very dry skin you can add a teaspoon of olive or other massage oil, although it will decrease the bubbly effect of the potion.

The Face

Essentials oils can protect the skin from damage and promote circulation and new cell growth. Rosemary is very high in antioxidants, and lavender is good for just about everything, but it has shown to improve skin regeneration and prevent scarring. Rose and frankincense are excellent for wrinkles and age spots and are gentle to the skin.

Individual essential oils can be moisturizing or drying for oily skin. Here are some great recipes.

Tightener

2 teaspoons hydrated bentonite clay   1 teaspoon Moor mud
1 teaspoon witch hazel   1 egg, lightly beaten
5 drops lavender essential oil   2 drops thyme linalool

This is more for oily skin. Mix it all together and let dry about 10 minutes, then rinse with cool water and pat skin dry. Follow with a good lotion potion.

Clear Skin

½ teaspoon hydrated bentonite   1 teaspoon Moor mud
1 teaspoon honey   1 drop rosemary
1 drop pink grapefruit   1 drop Helichrysum
2 capsules Proactazyme (NSP enzyme product)
Combine and let dry on face for 10 minutes, then rinse.

Toners

8 oz purified water   2 drops lavender
1 drop geranium   1 drop bergamot

For oily skin, use 6 oz distilled water, 3 drops mandarin, 2 drops lemon and 1 tablespoon witch hazel, but stay out of the sun! Keep in glass bottle and shake well before each use. Pour some on to a cotton ball and wipe face.

Cool Summer Spritzer's

2 ounce glass bottle with mister top   1 ¾ ounce of purified water
10-30 drops various essential oils   ¼ teaspoon vodka or witch hazel

Fill bottle with water and oils and shake well before each use.

Try these others:
Uplifting: 8 pink grapefruit, 3 mandarin, 2 neroli
Comforting: 4 lavender, 2 geranium, 1 chamomile
Tranquil: 5 bergamot, 3 marjoram, 3 lavender
Stimulating: 8 lemon, 4 pine, 2 frankincense
Fiery: 2 cinnamon, 1 clove, 2 mandarin
Citrus: 5 grapefruit, 2 mandarin, 2 lemon

An Amazing Body Wrap!

Well, if you can't make it into my office for a detox wrap, this is the next best thing! This amazing wrap can help detoxify and re-mineralize the largest organ of the body. We call it the skin.

A dry skin brush	2 cups Moore mud or hydrated bentonite
½ cup ground kelp	¼ cup ground dulse
1 lemon	½ cup warm aloe vera juice
Gauze	Old towels.

10-20 drops total of your choice essential oils, using the recipes above, or create you own.

Combine dulse and kelp with the Moore mud or hydrated bentonite. Mix in the juice of half of the lemon, the essential oils, and as much aloe vera juice as needed to make a smooth paste. Dry skin brush your skin, starting at your feet and working toward the heart, one leg at a time. Smear the mixture over your skin and wrap with gauze, as soon as your leg is covered. Continue until your entire body is covered, with the exception of your face. (If you want, do a light facemask at the same time.) Light a fragrant candle, lie back in the tub and cover yourself in the towels or sheets. Listen to some positive affirmations you have prerecorded onto a tape, or play some soothing music. After 20 minutes, remove the gauze, and quickly shower. Do not use this recipe if you are allergic to iodine or seaweed.

Cellulite
For extra attention to cellulite areas, combine more of the grapefruit, geranium, rosemary, thyme linalool, cypress, juniper, niaouli, vetiver and 3 drops peppermint with ¼ cup aloe vera juice (do not use aloe vera "gel" unless you are going to use a pour bottle. In this case you can add 3 teaspoons massage oil, right into the bottle.) Otherwise, add ½ teaspoon vodka or witch hazel to a glass spritzer bottle, half full of mineral water. Shake well and spritz lightly over affected areas. Add a few drops jojoba oil to hands and knead into skin, twice daily. Drink plenty of water and add vitamin C and E to the diet, as well.

Hair
You can use your regular shampoos and just add your essential oils right to the bottles. Test for sensitivity to oils before using. For an overnight treatment your scalp will love you for, try this recipe:

2 drops lavender	2 drops rosemary
3 drops thyme linalcol	1 teaspoon jojoba oil

Combine these oils in a shot glass and place in a pot of warm water. Once the mixture is warm, apply directly to scalp and allow to sit overnight on scalp. In the morning, wash hair as usual and rinse with 1 cup apple cider vinegar, diluted with ½ cup water. This recipe can help reduce the amount of Falling hair!

Cleaning Your House with Essential Oils

Disinfecting Laundry Freshener

7 drops tea tree
5 drops Lavender
3 drops thyme
2 drops rosemary
7 drops lemon
2 drops pine needle

Mix essential oils with ¼ tsp castile soap then add to laundry while basin is filling but before clothes are loaded. Be sure to dry your cloths completely afterwards.

Disinfectant Spray for Surfaces

3 drops cinnamon leaf
5 drops pine needle
2 drops frankincense
10 drops bergamot
1/4 teaspoon liquid castile soap
2 oz purified water

Combine essential oils with soap in a trigger spray bottle. Spray on countertops, stove tops, and tile, then wipe surface dry.

Disinfecting Floor Cleaner

1 tablespoon castile soap
11 drops lemon

3 drops eucalyptus
4 drops pink grapefruit
7 drops peppermint

While filling a bucket with very warm water, add the soap and essential oils. Mop up the floors, tile and countertops and breathe deep the wonderful fragrance!

Natural Surface Scrubber

Turn any of these essential oils into a safe surface scrub for your sinks, tub, shower & floors.
2 tablespoons of baking soda
2 teaspoons castile soap
7-10 drops of your favorite essential oil

Mix it into a thick paste and scrub. Be sure to rinse afterwards.

♥ Safe Ingredient Handling Tips

These tips are designed to help you create your products safely. The concentrated active ingredients which you may be working with are usually diluted, for safe consumer use. These ingredients which benefit consumers may create problems for you.

Good Manufacturing Practices (GMP) will help you control the quality of your products. Basically GMP's are a system of record keeping and written procedures to ensure consistency. Lot #s and records can help you trouble-shoot your products. They can also help recover products, if a recall is needed. Be sure to follow directions carefully.

When experimenting on your own, be sure to document your recipes and ingredient mixtures, in case of an allergic reaction. Here are some guidelines to help you enjoy your products safely.

1) Wear safety glasses to protect your eyes. Active essential oils are readily absorbed through the eyes and skin.

2) Get professional advice before applying ANY essential oil to your body or anyone else.

3) Use extra caution if you are pregnant.

4) Use pot holders when working with heated glass and pots. Remember, hot oils can cause severe burns.

5) Wear an apron and wash it regularly. If your clothes don't get dirty, you won't. Keep hair tied back, away from flames. Think about your procedures to ensure that they are safe. Keep your work area clean and sterile.

6) Prevent skin irritation and absorption of active essential oils and preservatives. Wear gloves and change them regularly.

7) Use separate utensils from food utensils to measure lye, essential oils, and preservatives. Use larger bowls and buckets to mix even smaller batches.

8)   Know the properties and precaution for the essential oils you use. Things like Citronella and dl-Limonene-based products should not be used on cats. Ask for books that describe the properties of essential oils before you use them.

9)   Label your products for consumer safety, even if they are home made gifts. It's an FDA requirement. Label your mixing containers as you use them to ensure that no one will mistake them for food and be injured.

10)   Be careful when you melt solid oils. They can be persuaded to burn, with extended direct heating. Keep baking soda or a fire extinguisher near.

11)   Powdered materials (citric acid, clay, lye) can be lung irritants, or worse. Wear a mask to measure and sift dry ingredients. Keep the dust down and work in a well-ventilated area.

12)   Get a Material Safety Data Sheet (MSDS) for every product that you use. Read them, especially the health warnings and safety precautions. Keep all your MSDS in a book. OSHA requires it and doctors can't treat without it. Show this book to anyone who may come in contact with the products.

13)   Test your products for sterility and keep good records. Again, think about your procedures to ensure that they are safe.

14)   If you are making kits, products, and potions at home, be sure your environment is secure (kids, dogs, unexpected guests, etc.) before you begin, and be sure to store ALL your products out of the reach of children and keep all instructional and safety materials with the products.

♥ These guidelines are lovingly offered to help you safely create
Self♥Love Potions. ♥

♥This Herbalist's Library.

♥I found my personal library dwindling in size over the years, so I asked my assistant to take an inventory of the books that were left. I figured this way I could keep better track of the books I was lending out to patients and friends, and be sure they were returned. However, the lists kept disappearing faster than the books could be listed.

I couldn't figure out why anyone would want my lists. Then it was brought to my attention that people who liked the information I was offering them seemed to want more of the same, and a list of books from my personal library might give one a peek into the history of my learning. Who knows? So, I made up several copies and our patients went wild for it.

So, for what it's worth to you, I have included a portion of that list here in the bibliography. Some books were certainly more insightful and inspiring to me than others. Some I found to be worth little more than the paper they were printed on. In any case, I believe education (it matters little whether it is self-education or formal education) remains the single most empowering healing tool we have available to us today.

> ♥That includes the education and discovery of information we choose to reject. ♥

> ♥That includes the education and discovery of information we choose to reject. ♥

The truth is always available to us. The question is: How hard are we willing to work to discover it? A patient once asked me which single book I would choose from this list if I were to be stranded on a desert island for thirty years. Know what my answer was? *The Inspirational Bible* by Max Lucado.

Yup. The Bible. No, not just for its Spiritual value. I would choose it because it is such a great user's manual for the human body; a romantic novel; a relationship guide, an inspirational survival training guide, and an all around great mystery.

What would your answer be? Why not take an inventory of your own personal library? Add a few new books or lend a few out. You may even find a great treasure you'll want to read and re-read again and then share with a friend. Enjoy!

Bibliography

(Various). *An assortment of various bibles & study books*

Abanes, Richard. *Embraced by the Light and the Bible*. Camp Hill, PA: Horizon Books, 1994.

Airola Ph.D, Paavo. *How to Get Well*. Sherwood Oregon: Health Plus 1974.

Alexander, Scott. *Advanced Rhinocerology*. Laguna Hills, CA: The Rhino's Press, 1981.

Alexander, Scott. *Rhinoceros Success*. Laguna Hills CA: The Rhino's Press, 1980.

Alexander, Scott. *Rhinocerotic Relativity*. Laguna Hills, CA: The Rhino's Press Inc., 1983.

Allen, Dr. Patricia. *Staying Married and Loving It*. New York, New York: William Morrow and Co., 1997.

Allen, Patricia and Harmon, Sandra. *Staying Married and Loving It*. New York, NY: William Morrow and Company, Inc., 1997.

Andrecht, Venus Catherine. *The Outrageous Herb Lady*. Ramona CA: Ransom Hill Press, 1990.

Andrews, Ted. *Animal Speak*. St. Paul MN: Llewellyn Publications, 2001.

Andrews, Ted. *How to See and Read the Aura*. St. Paul MN: Llewellyn Publications, 1997.

Angier, Natalie. *Woman*. New York New York: Anchor Books, 1999.

Arthur, Kay. *A Marriage Without Regrets*. Eugene OR: Harvest House Publishers, 2000.

Bach, Marcus. *The Chiropractic Story*. Austell, GA: Si-Nel Publishing and Sales Co., 1968.

Bach, Richard. *Illusions*. New York NY: Dell Publishing, 1977.

Backus, William. *Finding the Freedom of Self-Control.* Minneapolis, MN: Bethany House Publishers, 1987.

Balch, CNC, Phyllis and Balch, M.D., James F. *Prescription for Nutritional Healing.* New York NY: Penguin Putnam Inc., 2000.

Balch, M. D., James F. *Prescription for Natural Healing.* Garden City Park, NY: Avery Publishing Group Inc., 1990.

Barbach, PhD., Lonnie. *The Pause.* New York, NY: Penguin Group, 1993.

Black, Dean. *Health at the Crossroads. Springville.* Springville UT: Tapestry Press, 1988.

Block, Ph.D., Joel D. *Secrets of Better Sex.* West Nyack NY: Parker Publishing Co. 1996.

Boutenko, Victoria. *12 Steps to Raw Foods.* Ashland, OR: Raw Family Publishing, 2000.

Brady, Joan. *God on a Harley.* New York NY: Pocket Books, 1995.

Brennan, Barbara Ann. *Hands of Light.* New York NY: Bantam Books, 1987.

Brown M.D., Rebecca. *Prepare for War.* Springdale PA: Whitaker House, 1987.

Browne, Sylvia. *Life on the Other Side.* New York NY: The Penguin Group, 2000.

Bryan, Mark. *The Prodigal Father.* New York NY: Three River Press, 1997.

Campbell, Don. *The Mozart Effect.* New York New York: Avon Books, Inc., 1997.

Canfield, Jack and Hansen, Mark Victor. *Chicken Soup for the Soul.* Deerfield Beach, FL: Health Communications, Inc., 1993.

Cantwell, JR., M. D. Alan. *AIDS The Mystery & The Solution.* Los Angeles, CA: Aries Rising Press, 1983.

Carlson M.D., Dwight L. *Overcoming Hurts and Anger.* Eugene OR: Harvest House Publishers, 1981.

Carlson, Ph.D., Richard. *Don't Worry Make Money.* New York NY: Hyperion, 1998.

Carter, Dr. Les. *Imperative People.* Nashville, TN: Thomas Nelson Inc., 1991.

Cerney, J. V. *Acupuncture without Needles.* Parker Publishing Co. Inc., 1974.

Cheraskin, M.D., D.M.D., and Ringsdorf, Jr. D.M.D., and Clark, D.D.S, *Diet and Disease.* New Canaan, Connecticut: Keats Publishing, Inc., 1968.

Chopra, Deepak. *How to Know God.* New York New York: Harmony Books, 2000

Chopra, M. D., Deepak. *Perfect Health.* New York, NY: Harmony Books, 1991.

Cianciosi, John. *The Meditative Path.* Wheaton IL: Quest Books, 2001.

Cole, Henri. *The Look of Things.* New York NY: Alfred A. Knopf, Inc., 1994.

Colgan, Dr. Michael. *Hormonal Health.* Vancouver, British Colombia: Apple Publishing, 1996.

Collier Cool, Lisa. *How to Write Irresistible Query Letters.* Cincinnati OH: Writer's Digest Books, 1987.

Crenshaw, M.D., Theresa L. *The Alchemy of Love and Lust.* New York NY: Pocket Books, 1996.

Cunningham, Scott. *Cunningham's Encyclopedia of Magical Herbs.* St. Paul MN: Llewellyn Worldwide, 2000.

Cunningham, Scott. *Earth, Air, Fire, and Water.* St. Paul MN: Llewellyn Publications, 2000.

Cunningham, Scott. *Wicca.* St. Paul MN: Llewellyn Publications, 2000.

Curtis, Bud. *Remove the Thorn & God Will Heal.* Victorville, CA: Curtis, 1993.

Cypert, Samuel A. *The Power of Self-Esteem*. New York, NY: Amacom, 1994.

DeGoede, PhD., Daniel L. and Drews, C.A.S., Danae. *Belief Therapy*. Lake Elsinore CA: E.D.L. Productions, 1998.

Densmore, Frances. *How Indians Use Plants for Food, Medicine and Crafts*. New York NY: Dover Publications, Inc.

Dobson, Dr. James. *The New Dare to Discipline*. Wheaton, IL: Tyndale Publishing, Inc., 1970.

Dockrey, Karen. *Spiritual Gifts*. Colorado Springs CO: WaterBrook Press, 1999.

Dossey, M. D., Larry. *Space, Time and Medicine*. Boston MA Shambhala Publications Inc, 1982.

Douglass, M. D., William Campbell. *AIDS: The End of Civilization*. Brooklyn, NY: A&B Books Publishers, 1989.

Dumas, Alexander. *The Count of Monte Cristo*. New York: The Modern Library, 1996.

Elliot, Elisabeth. *Passion and Purity*. Grand Rapids Michigan: Fleming H. Revell, 1984.

Farrar, Mary. *Choices*. Siters, OR: Multnonah Books, 1994.

Fast, Julius. *Body Language*. New York, NY: MJF Books, 1970.

Feldhahn, Shaunti Christine. *Y2K*. Sisters OR: Multnomah Publishers, 1998.

Finney, John. *Saints Alive!* Derby, London: Anglican Renewal Ministries, 1992.

Ford, Charlotte. *Ford's Etiquette*. New York NY: Clarkson N. Potter, Inc. Publishers, 1988.

Foster, Richard J. *Coming Home*. New York NY: HarperSanFrancisco, 1992.

Foundation for Inner Peace. *A Course in Miracles*. Glen Ellen, CA: Foundation for Inner Peace, 1975

Freud, Sigmund. *The Interpretation of Dreams*. New York, NY: Random House Inc., 1950.

Gawain, Shakti. *Meditations.* San Rafael, CA: New World Library, 1991.

Gerber, Michael E. *The E Myth Revisited.* New York, NY: Harper Collins Publishers Inc., 1995.

Glenmullen, M.D., Joseph. *Prozac Backlash.* New York NY: Simon and Schuster, 2000.

Goldberg, Ph.D., Marilee C. *The Art of the Question.* New York: John Wiley and Sons, 1998.

Goulston, Mark and Goldberg, Philip. *Get Out Of Your Own Way.* New York, NY: The Berkley Publishing Group, 1996.

Gray, Alice. *Stories for the Heart.* Gresham, OR: Vision House Publishing Inc., 1996.

Gray, Ph.D., John. *Mars and Venus on a Date.* New York NY: HarperPerennial, 1997.

Gray, PhD., John. *Mars & Venus Starting Over.* New York, NY: Harper Collins Publishers, 1998.

Griggs, Barbara. *The Green Witch Herbal.* Rochester VT: Healing Arts Press, 1994.

Grof, M.D., Stanislav. *Spiritual Emergency.* New York NY: G.P. Putnam's Sons, 1989.

Halfmoon, PhD., Hygeia. *Primal Mothering in a Modern World.* San Diego, CA: Maul Brothers Publishing, 1998.

Harrar, Sari, and Vantine, Julia. *Extraordinary Togetherness.* Emmaus, Pennsylvania: Rodale Press Inc., 1999.

Hawken, C. M. *Parasites.* UT: Woodland Pub., 1997.

Hiam, Alexander and Lewicki, Roy J. *The Fast Forward MBA in Negotiating and Deal Making.* New York NY: John Wiley and Sons, Inc., 1999.

Higley, Connie and Allen. *Quick Reference Guide for Using Essential Oils.* Olathe, KS: Abundant Health, 1998.

Hoffer, M.D., Ph.D., Abram and Walker, D.P.M., Morton. *Putting it All Together: The New Orthomolecular Nutrition*. New Cannan, Connecticut: Keats Publishing, Inc., 1978.

Hoffman, David. *Holistic Herbal*. Boston, MA: Element Books Limited, 1996.

Holloway, Jr., William D. and Joiner-Bey, N.D., Herb. *Water*. New York NY: Impakt Health, 2002.

Hopkins, Tom. *How to Master the Art of Selling*. Scottsdale, AZ: Tom Hopkins Intl. Inc., 1982.

Jacoby, Russell. *Dogmatic Wisdom*. New York, NY: Doubleday, 1994.

Janov, Dr. Arthur. *The Biology of Love*. Amherst NY: Prometheus Books, 2000.

Jeffress, Robert. *Coming Home to the Father Who Loves You*. Sisters OR: Multnomah Books, 1997.

Jenks, James. *Herb Power*. NV: J Pub., 1996.

Jensen, Bernard. *A Hunza Trip*. Escondido, CA: Jensen Ent., 1938.

Jensen, Bernard. *A New Lifestyle for Health & Happiness*. Escondido, CA: Jensen Ent., 1980.

Jensen, Bernard. *Arthritis, Rheumatism & Osteoporosis*. Escondido, CA: Jensen Ent., 1986.

Jensen, Bernard. *Bee Well-Bee Wise*. Escondido, CA: Jensen Ent., 1994.

Jensen, Bernard. *Chlorella, Jewel of the Far East*. Escondido, CA: Jensen Ent., 1992.

Jensen, Bernard. *Color, Music & Vibration*. Escondido, CA: Jensen Ent., 1988.

Jensen, Bernard. *Creating a Magic Kitchen*. Escondido, CA: Jensen Ent., 1973.

Jensen, Bernard. *Doctor-Patient Handbook*. Escondido, CA: Jensen Ent., 1976.

Jensen, Bernard. *Love, Sex & Nutrition*. Garden City Park, NY: Avery Publishing Group Inc., 1988.

Jensen, Bernard. *Master Feeding Program.* Escondido, CA: Jensen Ent., 1988.

Jensen, Bernard. *Nutrition Handbook.* Escondido, CA: Jensen Ent., 1993.

Jensen, Bernard. *Nutrition Handbook.* Escondido, CA: Jensen Ent., 1993.

Jensen, Bernard. *Soil & Immunity.* Escondido, CA: Jensen Ent., 1988.

Jensen, Bernard. *Survive This Day.* Escondido, CA: Jensen Ent., 1976.

Jensen, Bernard. *The Greatest Story I've Ever Told.* Escondido, CA: Jensen Ent., 1988.

Jensen, Bernard. *The Healing Power of Chlorophyll from Plant Life.* Escondido, CA: Jensen Ent., 1984.

Jensen, Bernard. *Unfoldment of the Great Within.* Escondido, CA: Jensen Ent., 1992.

Jensen, Bernard. *What is Iridology?* Escondido, CA: Jensen Ent., 1984.

Jensen, Bernard. *Your Home for Health, Happiness & Fitness.* Escondido, CA: Jensen Ent., 1996.

Jensen, D.C. Ph.D., Bernard. *The Healing Power of Chlorophyll.* Escondido CA: Bernard Jensen Enterprises, 1973.

Jensen, Karen A. *Nature Makes Whole.* Provo, UT: Starbuck Co., 1988.

Johnson, Denny. *What the Eye Reveals.* Goleta, CA: Rayid Publications, 1984.

Kershaw, Linda. *Edible & Medicinal Plants of the Rockies.* Renton, WA: LonePine Publishing, 2000.

Kroeger, Hanna. *Parasites: The Enemy Within.* Hanna Kroeger Publications, 1991.

Kuck, Sandra. *Angel Kisses.* Eugene OR: Harvest House Publishers, 2000.

Kuhatschek, Jack. *Spiritual Welfare.* Downers Grove Il: InterVarsity Press, 1999.

Kunz, Barbara and Kevin. *The Complete Guide to Foot Reflexology.* Albuquerque NM: Kunz and Kunz, 1993.

LaHaye, Tim and Jenkins, Jerry B. *Apollyon.* Wheaton Illinois: Tyndale House Publishers, Inc., 1999.

LaHaye, Tim and Jenkins, Jerry B. *Assassins.* Wheaton Illinois: Tyndale House Publishers, Inc., 1999.

LaHaye, Tim and Jenkins, Jerry B. *Left Behind.* Wheaton Illinois: Tyndale House Publishers, Inc., 1995.

LaHaye, Tim and Jenkins, Jerry B. *Nicolae.* Wheaton Illinois: Tyndale House Publishers, Inc., 1997.

LaHaye, Tim and Jenkins, Jerry B. *Soul Harvest.* Wheaton Illinois: Tyndale House Publishers, Inc., 1998.

LaHaye, Tim and Jenkins, Jerry B. *Tribulation Force.* Wheaton Illinois: Tyndale House Publishers, Inc., 1996.

Lama, Dalai. *The Art of Happiness.* New York NY: Riverhead Books, 1998.

Lark, M. D., Susan M. *The Estrogen Decision.* Los Altos, CA: Westchester Publishing Co., 1994

Laurie, Greg. *God's Design for Christian Dating.* Eugene OR: Harvest House Publishers, 1983.

Lepore, N.D., Donald. *The Ultimate Healing System.* Woodland Publishing Inc., 1985.

Levine, Mark and Pollan, Stephen M. *Live Rich.* New York NY: HarperBusiness, 1998.

Lewis, James R. and Oliver, Evelyn Dorothy. *Angels A to Z.* Detroit, Michigan: Visible Ink Press, 1996.

Lininger, Schuyler. *A-Z Guide to Drug-Herb-Vitamin Interactions.* Roseville, CA: Prima Publishing, 1999.

Louden, Jennifer. *The Woman's Retreat Book.* New York NY: HarperCollins Publishers, 1997.

Lynch, Jerry and Chungliang, Al Huang. *Working Out, Working Within.* New York, NY: Penguin Putnam, 1998.

Macpherson, David. *Change Your Attitude.* Newport Beach CA: MacBay Presentations, 1997.

Malstrom, N. D., Stan. *Natural Approach To Female Problems.* Orem, UT: BiWorld Publishers, 1997.

Martinet, Jeanne. *The Art of Mingling.* New York NY: St Martin's Press, 1992.

Martlew, N.D., Gillian. *Electrolytes the Spark of Life.* Murdock FL: Nature's Publishing, Ltd., 1994.

McGraw, Ph.D., Phillip C. *Self Matters.* New York NY: Simon and Schuster Source, 2001.

Melcombe, Lynne. *Health Hazards of White Sugar.* Vancouver, Can: Alive Books, 2002.

Mickaharic, Draja. *Spiritual Cleansing.* Yourk Beach, Me: Samuel Weiser Inc., 1982.

Mindell, Earl L. PhD. *The MSM Miracle.* CT: Keats Publishing, 1997.

Mindell, Earl. *Vitamin Bible.* New York, NY: Warner Books, 1991.

Moore, Thomas. *Care of the Soul.* New York NY: HarperPerennial, 1992.

Morter, Dr. M. Ted, *Your Health Your Choice.* Hollywood, FL: Lifetime Books Inc., 1995.

Mowrey, PhD., Daniel B. *The Scientific Validation Of Herbal Medicine.* New Canaan, CT: Keats Pub. Inc., 1986.

Mullins, Eustace. *Murder by Injection.* Stauanton, Virginia: Mullins, 1988.

Muncaster, Ralph O. *How Is Jesus Different from Other Religious Leaders?* Eugene, OR: Harvest House Publishers, 2001.

Muncaster, Ralph O. *What Really Happens When You Die?* Eugene, OR: Harvest House Publishers, 2000.

Murray, Michael T. *Chronic Fatigue Syndrome* Rocklin, CA: Prima Publishing, 1994.

Nair, Ken. *Discovering the Heart of a Man.* Phoenix, AZ: Nair, 1986.

Nerburn, Kent. *The Wisdom of the Native Americans.* Novato, CA: New World Library, 1999.

Omartian, Stormie. *Just Enough Light for the Step I'm On.* Eugene OR: Harvest House Publishers, 1999.

Omartian, Stormie. *The Power of a Praying Parent.* Eugene OR: Harvest House Publishers, 1995.

Omartian, Stormie. *The Power of a Praying Wife.* Eugene OR: Harvest House Publishers, 1997.

Orman, Susan. *The Courage to be Rich.* New York NY: Riverhead Books, 1999.

Ornstein, Robert E. *The Psychology of Consciousness.* New York, NY: Harcourt Brace Jovanovich, Inc., 1977.

Pearsall, PhD., Paul. *The Heart's Code.* New York, NY: Broadway Books, 1998.

Pederson, Mark. *Nutritional Herbology.* Ut: Pederson Publishing, 1987.

Peikin, Steven, *M. D., Gastrointestinal Health.* NY: Harper Perennial, 1992.

Penner, Ph.D., Clifford L. and Penner, M.N., R.N., Joyce J. *Men and Sex.* Nashville, Tennessee: Thomas Nelson, Inc., Publishers, 1997.

Peretti, Frank E. *This Present Darkness.* Wheaton IL: Crossway Books, 1986.

Pert, Ph.D., Candace B. *Molecules of Emotion.* New York NY: Simon and Schuster, 1997.

Phillips, Gerald M. *Help for Shy People.* New York, NY: Barnes & Nobel Books Inc., 1981.

Piven, Joshua and Borgenicht, David. *The Worst Case Scenario Survival Handbook.* San Francisco CA: Chronicle Books, 2001.

Pliner Rodnitzky, Donna. *Ultimate Jucing.* Roseville CA: Prima Health, 2000.

Ponder, Catherine. *Open Your Mind to Prosperity.* Marina Del Ray, CA: DeVorss & Co. Publisher, 1971.

Pressman, David. *Patent it Yourself.* Berkley CA: Nolo Press, 1985.

Price, Shirley and Price Parr, Penny. *Aromatherapy for Babies and Children.* San Francisco CA: Thorsons, 1996.

Prophet, Elizabeth Clare. *The Creative Power of Sound.* Corwin Springs, MT: Summit University Press, 1998.

Prophet, Mark L. and Prophet, Elizabeth Clare. *Creative Abundance.* Corwin Springs MT: Summit University Press, 1998.

Ramirez Basco, Ph.D., Monica. *Never Good Enough.* New York NY: The Free Press, 1999.

Ridenour, Fritz. *So What's the Difference?.* Ventura CA: Regal, 1973.

Robbins, Anthony. *Unlimited Power.* New York, NY: Ballantine Books, 1986.

Robinson, L. Carl. *The Scents of Health.* Roosevelt, UT: Tree of Light Institute, Inc, 1998.

Roget, Peter Mark. *Roget's Thesaurus.* Ottenheiner Publishers Inc., 1972.

Roueche, Berton. *The Medical Detectives.* New York, NY: The Penguin Group, 1947.

Ruiz, Don Miguel. *The Four Agreements.* San Rafael, CA: Amber Allen Publishing Inc., 1997.

Russell, Rex. *What the Bible Says About Healthy Living.* Ventura California: Regal Books, 1996.

Sandler, David H. *You Can't Teach a Kid to Ride a Bike at a Seminar.* New York NY: The Penguin Group, 1995.

Schierse Leonard, Linda. *The Wounded Woman.* Boston, Massachusetts: Shambhala Publications , Inc , 1982.

Schiller, David and Carol. *500 Formulas for Aromatherapy.* New York, NY: Sterling Publishing Co. Inc., 1994.

Schlessinger, Dr. Laura. *How Could You Do That?!.* New York, NY: Harper Collins, 1996.

Schlessinger, Dr. Laura. *Ten Stupid Things Women Do to Mess Up Their Lives.* New York NY: HarperPerennial, 1994.

Schlosser, Eric. *Fast Food Nation.* New York NY: Houghton Mifflin Company, 2001.

Schuller, Robert H. *Prayer: My Soul's Adventure with God.* Nashville, TN: Thomas Nelson Inc., 1995.

Schuller, Robert. *Power Thoughts.* New York NY: HarperCollins Publishers, Inc., 1993.

Sears, PhD., Barry. *Enter The Zone.* New York, NY: Regan Books, 1995.

Simmons, Barbara & Lee. *Penny Pinching.* New York, NY: Bantam Books, 1991.

Sonberg, Lynn. *The Complete Nutrition Counter.* New York NY: Berkley Books, 1993.

Spieker, Michelle Morris. *The Cherished Self.* San Juan Capistrano, CA: Quality Books, Inc., 2000.

Stevens, M.D., David. *Jesus M.D.* Grand Rapids, Michigan: Zondervan Publishing House, 2001.

Steward, and Betha, M.D., Morrison C. and Andrews, M.D., Sam S., and Balart, M.D., Luis A. *Sugar Busters.* New York NY: Ballantine Books, 1995.

Stowell, Joseph M. *The Weight of Your Words.* Chicago IL: Moody Press, 1998.

Stoycoff, Cheryl. *Raw Kids.* Somerset, CA: Living Spirit Press, 2000.

Tenney, M. H., Louise. *Health Handbook.* Provo, UT: Woodland Books, 1987.

Thompson, George. *Verbal Judo.* New York, NY: William Morrow, 1993.

Tierra, C.A., N.D., Michael. *Planetary Herbology.* Twin Lakes, Wisconsin: Lotus Press, 1988.

Tolle, Eckhart. *The Power of Now.* Novato CA: New World Library, 1999.

Trent, John and Smalley, Gary. *The Blessing.* New York, NY: Pocket Books, 1979.

Vanzant, Jyanla. *One Day My Soul Just Opened Up.* New York NY: Fireside, 1998.

Victoria. *Bath and Beauty.* New York NY: Hearst Books, 1998.

Vincent Peale, Norman. *A Guide to Confident Living.* Avenel NJ: Prentice-Hall, 1948.

Vincent Peale, Norman. *The Tough-Minded Optimist.* New York : Balantine Books, 1961.

Virtue, Doreen. *Angel Therapy.* Carlsbad, CA: Hay House Inc., 1997.

Virtue, Ph.D., Doreen. *Divine Prescriptions.* Los Angeles CA: Renaissance Books, 2000.

Warren, Ph.D., Neil Clark. *Learning to Live With the Love of Your Life.* Wheaton IL: Tyndale House Publishers, 1995.

Warren, Rick. *The Purpose Driven Church.* Grand Rapids Michigan: Zondervan Publishing House, 1995.

Webster. *New Webster's Spanish-English Dictionary.* Miami, FL: Paradise Press Inc., 1994.

Weed, Susan S. *Menopausal Years.* Woodstock NY: Ash Tree Publishing, 1992.

Weed, Susan S. *Wise Woman Herbal for the Childbearing Year.* Woodstock NY: Ash Tree Publishing, 1986.

Wigmore, Ann. *The Wheatgrass Book.* Wayne, NJ: Avery Publishing Group Inc., 1985.

Wilkinson, Bruce. *Secrets of the Vine.* Sisters Oregon: Multnomah Publishers, Inc., 2001.

Wilkinson, Bruce. *The Prayer of Jabez.* Sisters OR: Multnomah Publishers, 2000.

Williamson, Marianne. *A Return To Love.* New York, NY: Harper Perennial, 1992.

Williamson, Marianne. *A Women's Worth.* New York, NY: Random House, 1993.

Worwood, Valerie Ann. *The Fragrant Mind.* Novato, CA: New World Library, 1996.

Wright, H. Norman. *Relationships That Work and Those That Don't.* Ventura CA: Regal, 1998.

Young, Ph.D., D.Sc., Robert O. *Sick and Tired?.* Pleasant Grove UT: Woodland Publishing, 2001.

Ziglar, Zig. *Over the Top.* Nashville, TN: Thomas Nelson, 1994.

♥ One Final Thought

Father, I ask you to bless the person who is reading this book, right now. I am asking You to minister to their Spirit, at this very moment. Where there is pain, provide peace and mercy. Where there is self-doubting, let go a renewed self-belief in Your ability to work through them. Where there is weariness or fatigue, I ask You to give them acceptance, tolerance, and power as they learn surrender to Your leading. Where there is Spiritual stagnation, I ask You to renew them by illuminating Your nearness, and draw them into greater intimacy with You. Where there is alarm, reveal Your love, and release to them Your courage. Where there is a sin blocking them, reveal it, and break its hold over their life. Bless their finances, give them a larger vision, and lift up friends to support and encourage them. Give them sensitivity to recognize the evil forces around them, and reveal to them the power they have in You to defeat them, completely! I want the person who reached for this book to see Your features in my expressions; because I love you, Father, and trust in Your promise to me; I ask You to do these things, in Jesus' name.

❤Resources:

Better Health Chiropractic & Cynthia's Self~Love Potions
28971 Golden Lantern Suite A102-103
Laguna Niguel, Ca. 92677
(949)481-9686
Website: www.selflovepotions.com
A Chiropractic & Natural Family health care center specializing in natural remedies and healthy living resources.
This is my office. (See back pages for more information.)

Nature's Sunshine Essential Oils and Herbal Products
Customer service 1800-223-8225
You will need a sponsor number to place a wholesale order. You can use our sponsor # 3472215 to get started and customer service will provide you with your own account number after that.
This company carries top of the line Natural Health Care products and essential oils, and they work hard to create easy-to-use educational materials to help you get started in natural healing, for yourself and your family, or to stimulate extra income, building a home-based business. I think this company is among the best for those just starting out in natural healing, especially busy moms. This is my personal favorite home-based business company because I love their customer service department. You may experience a three to five minute wait from time to time, however, once you know what you want, you can call order entry directly at 800-453-1422, and you will be greeted by some of the most knowledgeable, service-oriented employees I've ever encountered. They really pay attention to detail, truly listen to your complaints, and take action right away. You will love them!

Young Living Oils – Essential Oils and Herbal Products
Customer Service 1800 763-9963
You will need a sponsor number to place a wholesale order. Sponsor #148494
You may find complexity with their customer service department and calling in your orders takes a little extra patience and effort, but this company's combination oils can't be beat and may be worth the extra effort it takes to order them. I only use their combination oils, but they have a full line of other natural healing products as well.

❤Additional Resources:

Abundant Health
888-718-3068 www.abundant-health4u.com
11569 S. Burch Circle Olathe, KS 66061
A wonderful line of hard-to-find natural healing books, as well as those compatible with the Nature's Sunshine product line. Great for self-education, teaching classes in your home, and building a home-based business, using NSP products. They also have a wonderful line of inspirational greeting cards.

Abundant Life Seed Foundation
P.O. Box 772, Port Townsend, WA 98368
Herbal Seed Resource

Amaranthine Aromatics
www.amaranthine.com
A wonderful line of bottles, but you must buy in large quantities to get a good price break.

Blade
445 6th St., Brooklyn, NY 11215
Specializes in aphrodisiac products.

Boston Jojoba Company
800-2jOjOBA
P.O. Box 771, Middleton, MA 01949
Jojoba Oils

Dissatisfied Parents Together, Anti-Vaccination
800-909-7468 Web Site: www.909shot.com
Some interesting information every mom should consider.

Fedco Seeds
P.O. Box 520, Waterville, ME 04903
Herbal Seed Resource

Flowery Branch
P.O. Box 1330, Flowery Branch, GA 30542
Herbal Seed Resource

Get Fresh
+44 (0) 870-800-7070
Web Site: www.fresh-network.com

Healing Spirits
607-566-2701
9198 State Route 415, Avoca, NY f-14809
Family-run, organically grown dried herbs, beeswax and other herbal products.

Herb Pharm
503-846-7178
P.O. Box 116, Williams, OR, 97544
Wide-ranging line of herbal tinctures, compounds, salves, and liniments.

International Foundation for Homeopathy
4 Sherman Avenue
Fairfax, Ca. 90930

Just Eat an Apple Magazine
(800) 205-2350 Web Site www.nature@rawfood.com

Living Nutrition Magazine
707-887-9132 Web Site: www.livingnutrition.com

Mountain Rose Herbs
800-879-3337
85472 Dilley Lane, Eugene, OR 97405
I love this company! I can buy almost any item in small quantities. They offer a complete line of herbs, beeswax, carrier oils, jars, and containers. They also carry their own herbal body care products, face creams, hair products, books, and more.

Nature's First Law
619-645-7282
P.O. Box 900202 San Diego Ca. 92190
Web Site http//www.rawfood.com
Everything to do with every raw food book in print. Juicers, dehydrators, videos, audio tapes, and raw food items.

Northeast Herbal Association
P.O. Box 479, Milton, N.Y 12547
A networking and educational organization. Newsletters and directory.

Sensia.com
800-777-8027
Incense form India and Tibet.

Snowdrift Farm
888-999-6950
2750 South 4ᵗʰ Ave #107 Tucson AZ, 85713

This is a wonderful resource for bulk products as well as great recipes for lotions and body creams. Not all of their products are natural, but you can get hard-to-find supplies in bulk.

United Plant Savers
PO. Box 420, East Barret, VT 05649
A nonprofit organization for replanting and protecting endangered plants.

~A warm welcome awaits your arrival~

Cynthia is available for workshops, lectures, and private consultations. She is always happy to answer your general questions, whenever possible. Come in and meet our friendly staff, check out our retail center, or drop us an email with your requests at Charts2001@aol.com. For a complete list of additional services, please visit our website at www.selflovepotions.com or call our office at (949) 481-9686

Cynthia's in-office services available by appointment.

A Consultation

A consultation will certainly depend on your immediate needs, however, generally speaking, once you have made your appointment, you will be asked to keep a daily food and optional emotion log up until the time of your first visit. Once you arrive at Cynthia's office, you will be greeted by a smiling, friendly staff member, who will gather your information, and request that you fill out a basic health questionnaire and a nutrient survey. Cynthia will then invite you back to her office where a cushy, comfy, deep-set swiveling chair awaits your arrival. Once seated and relaxed, Cynthia will begin a physical, mental, emotional, and Spiritual evaluation, using a variety of non-invasive methods. Once the evaluation has been completed, Cynthia will provide you with a variety of options from which you may choose to help you reach your desired goals.

5 Day Miracle Detox

The decision to experience this 5-day detox is a commitment to your health now and in the future and will require sixty to ninety minutes to complete. Although visible results are immediate, I regularly see people making healthier lifestyle choices; mentally, emotionally and physically, with little desire to go back to their old habits because they feel so good after just one session! This is a great way to re kindle an already existing healthcare regimen or begin a new one. Your Consultation, 5-day Pre & Post Detox Herbal Supplements, Personalized Essential Oil, Dry Skin Brush, Oxygen Circulation Treatment, The Miracle Detox Body Wrap in our Self♥Love Room, 2 oz after-shower body lotion, and a 5-day easy-to-follow detox or weight loss strategy is included.

A Raindrop Experience
What is Raindrop, you ask? Simply speaking, it can be categorized as a massage. Raindrop therapy combines the ancient art of using essential oils for promoting health and well-being, with soothing touch, comforting sight, and peaceful sound. Essential oils are the vital life essences extracted from certain aromatic plants and flowers, and when properly combined and applied to specific areas of the body, they can be a very powerful Self-Love therapies, as well as an unbelievably peaceful experience. Each session lasts about forty-five minutes; I don't recommend you receive more than one session within a 4-week period.

Cynthia's Self♥Love Potion Products
Tell me your needs and I will create the perfect potion for you! No, it's not magic, silly! I use the ancient art of blending specific oils and herbs to capture their traditionally recognized energetic and medicinal properties. I have everything from bath soaks, salts and salves, to body lotions, oils and creams. I use only pure, 100% grade-A essential oils in all my products. Call me with your questions and I can create a potion perfect for you! They make great personal gifts!

The Self♥Loving Room
We read to figure out what is going on around us, but we write to figure out what is going on inside of us. I have found that (especially here in

fast-paced South Orange County) there is a need to just slow down and get out of our heads and rest the body so the heart and Spirit can do its healing job. I designed my balancing room for just that purpose. As you lie back on a magnetized mattress, you will find yourself soothed by the sound of trickling water as angels move peacefully behind the branches of a lush green forest tree. There is the cool element of an enchanted forest in the air as you stare up at the delicate fabric that drapes the ceiling, transforming the visual barrier into a limitless starry sky. As your feet are gently rocked back and forth by the steady movement of the "chi" machine, your mind drifts off to the visual pictures the guiding voice and music provides. After fifteen minuets of warmth upon a heated, magnetized mattress, you'll feel refreshed and awaken to eagerly answer the questions in your *Self-Love Potions* guide book, or write in your personal journal.

4-Week Clarity Sessions

This is the most popular 30-day plan. It is powerful and changes lives! It takes twenty-eight days to create a habit and it's going to take at least that long to create some new ones. This 4-week Clarity Session allows just enough time to offer you personal coaching techniques and the empowering choices life has to offer. Cynthia will see you twice a week for the first two weeks then once a week for the second two weeks. It includes one evaluation, two consultations, one essential oil, paraffin wax hand treatment, one Raindrop session, two Self-Love room sessions, suggestions for personal aroma therapy and herbal supplements, a workbook journal, goals board, weekly homework assignments and a nutrient survey. Order Cynthia's *Self-Love Potions* book directly from our website at www.selflovepotions.com, and show us your receipt for your full-price purchase and you will receive a $200.00 discount towards this 4-week session. Some restrictions may apply and offer may be rescinded without notice at any time

Monthly "Take Responsibility" Plan:
After an initial evaluation or following a 4-week Clarity Session, this plan is most helpful to keep a person grounded to their commitments for the next thirty days. It includes one Raindrop session and five Self-Love room journaling sessions (on your own) within a 30-day period of time.

0-595-23935-8

www.ingramcontent.com/pod-product-compliance
Lightning Source LLC
Chambersburg PA
CBHW061334280526
45784CB00001B/14